Shrink Rap

SHRINK

RAP

Three Psychiatrists Explain Their Work

Dinah Miller, M.D., Annette Hanson, M.D.,
and Steven Roy Daviss, M.D.

THE JOHNS HOPKINS UNIVERSITY PRESS

BALTIMORE

© 2011 Dinah Miller, Annette Hanson,
    Steven Roy Daviss
All rights reserved. Published 2011
Printed in the United States of America on
acid-free paper
9 8 7 6 5 4 3 2 1

The Johns Hopkins University Press
2715 North Charles Street
Baltimore, Maryland 21218-4363
www.press.jhu.edu

LIBRARY OF CONGRESS
CATALOGING-IN-PUBLICATION DATA

Miller, Dinah.
Shrink rap : three psychiatrists explain their work / Dinah Miller, Annette Hanson, and Steven Roy Daviss.
    p.   cm.
Includes index.
ISBN-13: 978-1-4214-0011-2 (hardcover : alk. paper)
ISBN-10: 1-4214-0011-1 (hardcover : alk. paper)
ISBN-13: 978-1-4214-0012-9 (pbk. : alk. paper)
ISBN-10: 1-4214-0012-X (pbk. : alk. paper)
1. Psychotherapy. 2. Psychotherapists. 3. Psychotherapy—Practice. I. Hanson, Annette. II. Daviss, Steven Roy. III. Title.
RC480.5.M533 2011
616.89'14—dc22   2010039015

A catalog record for this book is available from the British Library.

Special discounts are available for bulk purchases of this book. For more information, please contact Special Sales at 410-516-6936 or specialsales@press.jhu.edu.

The Johns Hopkins University Press uses environmentally friendly book materials, including recycled text paper that is composed of at least 30 percent post-consumer waste, whenever possible. All of our book papers are acid-free, and our jackets and covers are printed on paper with recycled content.

Contents

Introduction   1

A Note about Our "Patients" and Our "Doctors"   4

Chapter 1.
Melissa and Oscar: Getting Help   5

What are the different types of mental health professionals?
What is a psychiatrist?
What is a forensic psychiatrist?
When a patient should see a psychiatrist rather than
a primary care doctor
What is split treatment?
When a patient should see a psychiatrist for psychotherapy
When is split treatment better than care with only a psychiatrist?

Chapter 2.
Josh: A Walk through the System   21

The psychiatric evaluation and the mental status exam
The importance of outside informants
What is a chemical imbalance?
How psychiatric diagnoses are determined
Involuntary commitment to a psychiatric unit
What are a patient's rights during hospitalization?

Chapter 3.
The Brandt Family: Why People Seek Care   42

For psychiatric disorders
When life gets hard and stress causes symptoms
For psychiatric symptoms caused by medical illnesses
For maladaptive personality styles
For addictive or compulsive behaviors
For suicidal thoughts or behaviors
For insight and education

Chapter 4.
Tara: Let's Talk   61

What is psychotherapy?
What are some different types of psychotherapy?
How psychiatrists learn to become psychotherapists
How are research studies conducted on psychotherapy
      as a treatment?
What people talk about in psychotherapy
What the psychiatrist does in psychotherapy
Privacy and confidentiality in the therapeutic relationship:
      on keeping secrets and minding HIPAA
Special exceptions: child custody subpoenas and the Patriot Act
Self-disclosure by the therapist
How long should treatment last?

Chapter 5.
Josh Revisited: "Ask Your Doctor to Prescribe"   82

How psychiatric medications are (sort of) classified
How a doctor chooses a medication
Informed consent
Complementary and alternative treatments
How doctors dose medications
What happens when conventional treatments don't work?

Why psychiatrists don't like Xanax
Addictive medications in the treatment of the psychiatric patient

Chapter 6.
Becca: When Things Go Wrong 99

Difficulties with communication and poor patient-doctor fit
Recovered memory therapy
Disorders induced by the psychiatrist
When psychotherapy is inappropriately used as the only treatment
Side effects and adverse reactions from medications
Black box warnings
Antidepressants and suicide in young people and how the FDA
    decides on black box warnings
Boundary violations
Therapists who exploit patients

Chapter 7.
Eddie: A Child at Risk 122

Health care proxies, advance directives, and medical decision
    making for the dying patient
Informed consent and medical decisions for minors
Juvenile delinquency and the legal system
Custody evaluations: who gets the child?

Chapter 8.
Eddie: The Prison Patient 135

Specialty mental health courts and compelled treatment
Interrogation and why criminals confess
Psychopaths versus sociopaths and whether they can be treated
The insanity defense
What becomes of the insanity acquittee?
Psychiatric care in jail and in prison
Civil commitment of sex offenders

Chapter 9.
Mitchell: Hospital-based Psychiatry   158

What happens in the Emergency Department?
Finding a hospital bed for a psychiatric patient: insurance approval and bed availability
What happens during a psychiatric hospitalization?
Patient education, family involvement, and therapy
The agitated patient: restraint, seclusion, and forced medications
Shock treatments, or electroconvulsive therapy (ECT)
Bargaining for beds: insurance (again) and how psychiatric beds get allocated
Electronic health records
Day hospitals, or partial hospitalization programs
The consultation-liaison psychiatrist

Chapter 10.
Sharon: The Business of Psychiatry   183

Psychiatrists and insurance networks: how it all works
The missed appointment: no-shows and late cancellations
Preventing lawsuits
Providing safe environments for violent patients
When the patient assaults the psychiatrist
Changes in the patient's ability to pay for care
Influences of the pharmaceutical industry
Happy birthday! Gifts from patients

Chapter 11.
Things We Argue About   201

Health care reform and how we allocate our treatments   ·
What constitutes a psychiatric disorder: diagnostic criteria in the DSM age
Psychiatric disabilities and deciding who deserves special accommodation

Psychiatric disabilities in the workplace, from pilots to presidents
Medications with addictive potential
Medical marijuana for psychiatric disorders
Complementary and alternative treatments
The recovery model

Chapter 12.
The Future of Psychiatry   221

More than just medicines and psychotherapy: VNS, DBS,
    and rTMS
Just beginning: genetics, brain structure and function,
    and neuroplasticity
Psychopharmacogenetics: scientific gains that will lead
    to treatments based on each patient's biology

Acknowledgments   227

Sources and Suggested Reading   231

About the Authors   239

Index   247

Shrink Rap

Introduction

EVERY DAY, in many different settings, people seek out mental health services. Most do so voluntarily, but some who get care are required to—by the courts, by their employers, by their schools. Some patients come because they are desperate, others because they are curious. People want help with a wide range of problems. Some people have difficulties with their emotions, others have problems with their behaviors, some are plagued by unexplained physical symptoms, and some are temporarily overwhelmed by catastrophic life events. And finally there are those who want a better understanding of their own motivations, even if they aren't suffering from a mental illness.

What do psychiatrists think about when they approach a new patient? How do they decide what treatments to recommend? Psychiatric illnesses can be complicated. Many people have more than one mental illness, and mental illnesses can be caused or aggravated by medical illnesses and substance abuse. Treatments can be helpful or harmful, and not every patient has the same predictable pattern of illness, prognosis, or response to treatment. Because many symptoms of mental illness overlap with normal human emotions and behaviors, psychiatry becomes a natural target for controversy and is sometimes a muddle of disagreement.

Psychiatry can be seen as a mysterious and covert medical specialty. In part, this is due to the newness of the field and to the gaps in our knowledge about the definition, causes, and treatment of psychiatric disorders. This mystique is increased by the psychiatrist's traditional role as a psychotherapist who reveals little about himself and serves as a blank slate for patients—particularly psychoanalytic patients—to fill in with their own projections.

Patients come to treatment with unspoken expectations. Medicine, as a whole, has fostered a paternalistic approach to patient care, and psychiatric patients are often reluctant to question treatment recommendations. The intrigue is furthered by the confusion people have regarding what exactly psychiatrists do compared with other mental health professionals, or even compared with primary care physicians who prescribe psychotropic medications.

The psychoanalyst's couch has long been the icon for psychiatry. You'll find it in cartoons and movies, and people understand it to be an image for the field. Psychoanalysis, however, is a very small subspecialty of modern psychiatry—one that is steeped in mystery and that has its own theoretical ideologies. It is from psychoanalytic thought that we've grown to appreciate the construct of the unconscious, the idea that people's behavior may be motivated by their history, and the unique ways in which their minds deconstruct and reconstruct the events of their lives. Psychoanalytic theory has given us the concept of defense mechanisms—such as repression, projection, and denial—terms that have made their way easily into our everyday lives.

Psychoanalytic theory is also responsible for more complicated concepts that remain uncertain and elusive: the id, the ego, and the superego; pleasure and death principles; Oedipal complexes; and issues of infantile sexuality and psychosexual stages. Psychoanalytic theory has informed psychiatric thought for decades, and while its hypotheses remain largely unverifiable, it forms the basis for many of the newer psychotherapies. The treatment regimen for psychoanalysis, however, with the patient lying on the couch for four or five sessions a week, often for many years, has become impractical and inaccessible for most people.

In recent decades, we've refocused our understanding of psychiatric disorders toward more biological causes. The search is on to find the precise genes that determine mental illnesses and to find medications that lead to quicker and more reliable relief of suffering. Many would replace the image of the couch with an image of a brain, though neither fully captures what our field is all about.

As our understanding of psychiatric disorders has grown, we've also gained a greater appreciation for the legal and ethical implications of mental illness. Increasing numbers of psychiatric patients are being treated in forensic settings, and psychiatric training programs are now required to include education about the insanity defense, civil commitment, and patients' rights. Forensic, or legal, topics will be covered in some detail.

In *Shrink Rap*, we aim to demystify psychiatry and make it transparent by describing, in plain English, what we think about. We strive to avoid medical jargon and to communicate in a straightforward way about what we see, how we formulate patients' difficulties, and what treatments we have to offer.

Psychiatry remains full of shortcomings. We don't know what causes some people to become mentally ill while others remain well. We don't know why certain treatments work for one person while they make another person with the same condition even worse. Scientific studies have only begun to touch on what we need to know, and as individual practitioners, we often still struggle to diagnose and treat psychiatric problems. Our understanding of psychotherapy is inexact. The medication strategies we use are sometimes motivated by a desperate desire to help a tormented patient after the tested treatments have failed. There are so many more questions to ask and so few for which we have answers.

The shortcomings of our field notwithstanding, we hope you'll enjoy reading about our work as much as we enjoy doing it. Psychiatry has evolved a great deal over the past few decades, and we hope you'll find this journey into today's world of psychiatry illuminating.

A Note about Our "Patients" and Our "Doctors"

PSYCHIATRISTS STRUGGLE with how to write about their patients. On the one hand, case studies are essential to education. On the other hand, psychiatrists are obligated to keep their patients' secrets. It's not that clear how to write about an interesting "case." In academic journals, authors omit last names and obscure identifying information, but talking in detail about what has transpired in the privacy of a doctor-patient relationship remains both problematic and crucial. We have not been exempt from this struggle.

The patients in our book are fictional. We created them so that we could walk the reader through our professional lives in an interesting way. Because they are figments of our imagination, they represent typical patients. We avoided sensationalizing their symptoms. This book isn't about unusual syndromes; it's about what psychiatrists see in their everyday work lives. Using fictional patients freed us to write about what we do without the concern that our real patients might feel betrayed or wronged. Nonetheless, it seems odd to inject fictional people into a nonfiction book.

The psychiatrists are also fictional. As with their patient counterparts, we invented gestures, descriptions, and mannerisms for them. They react to their patients with specific thoughts and feelings. It's probably safe to assume that there is a little bit of us in these responses and reactions and that we've borrowed from our own internal lives to make our fictional psychiatrists all the more real.

Chapter 1

Melissa and Oscar:
Getting Help

MELISSA ADAMS is the nicest pediatrician a child could have. She softly sings the alphabet while examining a toddler and talks football draft picks with the teenage boys. She's an energetic woman with many friends and interests. Because Dr. Adams is such a vivacious person, people were shocked when she developed depression.

Everyone, even her patients' parents, asked Melissa if something was wrong. She could muster the energy to get to work, but she was irritable with her own family, and she lost interest in all the things she usually loved to do. She'd sneak off to the bathroom to cry during the workday. At night, she couldn't get settled in bed. She didn't return phone calls, and she skipped her high school reunion, even though she had helped organize it! Her husband insisted that something was wrong, and finally Melissa couldn't deny that she had depression, the mental illness she'd watched her father struggle with for years. She asked her internist to recommend a good psychiatrist—someone she didn't already know socially or professionally.

OSCAR FORD arrived in the emergency room in handcuffs. He was usually a charismatic man, but that night he was belligerent. The police brought him in after he was arrested for driving while intoxicated, something he hadn't done since he was a teenager. He'd told the arresting officer he was going to cut his wrists, so Oscar was brought to the hospital for an emergency psychiatric evaluation.

"You can't keep me here against my will. I *know* my rights! Now, get my clothes, goddamn it!" Oscar yelled.

He was a large and intimidating man, and he was very loud. However, he didn't really know his rights, and he could, indeed, be kept until he was not suicidal. Besides, he was under arrest. And because he was drunk, he'd later remember his behavior with a great deal of embarrassment.

A psychiatrist came to see Oscar in the Emergency Department. He learned that Oscar, an electrician, had separated from his wife six months ago and was in the middle of a custody battle for their two children. Oscar had always liked Guinness, but after his wife left, drinking it became a daily habit. Oscar also smoked a pack a day. He had health insurance, and he took medications for high blood pressure and high cholesterol. He'd never been arrested before, nor had he ever seen a psychiatrist.

Oscar had been feeling very depressed for several months. He cried often, slept poorly, and had lost fifteen pounds. He'd missed enough work to get a formal warning. He couldn't concentrate to read a newspaper, something he used to enjoy, and the papers had piled up on the front porch. He missed his wife, who'd left him for another man, and drinking dulled the loneliness. The night of the arrest, Oscar was supposed to have dinner with their children, but his wife refused to let the kids go with him. He went home and got drunk, then decided to drive back to her house. He was stopped by the police when his car started to swerve.

Neither Melissa Adams nor Oscar Ford is a real person. We invented them and their cases to walk through the process of how people realize they need mental health care and how they might go about getting it. Oscar may not be real, but his story is played out in every hospital emergency room every day. Suicidal people seek help regularly. Sometimes they are suicidal because they are suffering from mental illness, sometimes because they are distressed about a loss in their lives, and sometimes because they are intoxicated and make poor decisions. For Oscar Ford, it's a little of all three.

Melissa Adams's story is one that psychiatrists hear quite often. She has a genetic predisposition for a mood disorder, and she became depressed even though nothing specific triggered her depression. A physician herself, and the child of someone who suffered from major depression, she knows the symptoms of depression, and she knows how to negotiate the health care system.

One thing is clear here: both these patients need help. Many factors will determine how, where, and if they will get care, including their own beliefs about psychiatry, and what resources are available to them.

Oscar Ford needed immediate help. He was depressed, suicidal, and in police custody. He'd been brought to the hospital against his will, and in the emergency room he had his first encounter with mental health professionals. He was seen again in jail, and eventually a judge would mandate outpatient treatment as a condition of his release. Oscar Ford learned to navigate the mental health community.

Melissa Adams had an easier time getting help. She found it quietly and willingly, without so much fuss. She voluntarily sought a referral, made an appointment, and went to see a psychiatrist.

What are the different types of mental health professionals? Which professional should someone go to for treatment? And what exactly is a psychiatrist?

When a person thinks about a dentist, a specific image comes to mind. Perhaps it is of a man in a white coat standing over a patient in a reclining chair, and perhaps the dentist is saying, "Open wide." The image of an architect may be of someone hunched over detailed drawings of a building. What comes to mind when a psychiatrist is mentioned? Oscar Ford pictured a bearded man smoking a cigar, sitting behind a patient who is reclining on a couch. He was thinking of Sigmund Freud. Melissa Adams thought of a red-haired doctor in a white lab coat. She was thinking of the psychiatrist her father had seen at the university hospital for his depression. Both images may be accurate.

Psychiatrists may work with patients, or they may be involved in teaching, research, administration, or some combination of these. In this book, we are limiting our discussions to the *clinical* psychiatrist: one who works directly with patients for the purpose of providing treatment, rather than as part of a research protocol or for teaching purposes.

Psychiatrists are medical doctors (M.D.s) who specialize in illnesses that affect thoughts, emotions, perceptions, and behavior. These are brain-based disorders, but psychiatrists are not neurologists. Like all medical doctors, psychiatrists complete four years of college and four years of medical school. The first two years of medical school include two years of basic science followed by two years of clinical rotations through a variety of specialties, though the past decade has seen many programs develop a greater integration of clinical experiences within the initial basic science years. Every medical student does clerkships in medicine, surgery, pediatrics, neurology, obstetrics, and psychiatry. These clerkships last from one to three months, long enough to give each doctor a little experience in a range of specialties. After graduation from medical school, doctors train for several additional years as residents. A general psychiatric residency lasts four years. Subspecializations can be earned with further training during fellowships, which are typically one or two years. For example, child psychiatrists spend an additional one to two years in fellowship training. Other common fellowships include geriatrics, addiction, research, and psychosomatic medicine.

Psychiatrists diagnose and treat mental illnesses. They have the training necessary to make medication decisions and to prescribe medications, and although they are trained to perform several types of psychotherapy, they may or may not choose to focus on this. Some psychiatric residency programs emphasize psychotherapy training more than others, and factors that determine if a psychiatrist practices psychotherapy include the work setting, personal preference, and reimbursement issues. We talk about all these things in much more detail later.

Psychologists do not have medical training. They may have either a master's degree, in which case you'll see the initials M.A. or M.S. after their name, or they may have a doctoral degree, indicated by a Ph.D., Psy.D., or Ed.D. after their name. Only psychologists with doctoral degrees are called "doctor," though anyone with a doctoral degree in any subject can be called doctor. This is often confusing to many who limit their use of the term *doctor* to refer to medical physicians, such as psychiatrists and cardiologists.

Clinical social workers complete two years of graduate-level training to obtain a master's degree, or M.S.W. To receive the designation of *licensed* clinical social worker, or L.C.S.W., the therapist must have a period of clinical supervision and then pass a national exam. Social workers have no medical training and are not allowed to order diagnostic tests, administer psychological tests, or prescribe medications. In addition to therapy, the education of a clinical social worker involves learning how to provide for the financial and emotional needs of families and individuals by helping them obtain the programs and services they need.

While this seems clear enough, the distinctions can get very confusing. Some people have more than one degree, so that one person can conceivably be both a nurse and a social worker. Or a nurse can get a doctoral degree in nursing and be called doctor even though he's a nurse. Nurses can obtain a master's degree to provide psychotherapy, and in many states, licensed nurse practitioners and physicians' assistants can prescribe medications under loose supervision—"loose" meaning the supervising physician does not have to actually see the patient. A few states permit these health care providers to practice independently. The terms *counselor, therapist,* and *coach* may sometimes be used generically and not require any specific educational degree or licensure, though every state does things a little differently, so your mileage may vary. Being "certified" usually indicates less rigorous education and experience than being "licensed." The term *therapist* can refer to a psychiatrist, psychologist, social worker, nurse, or pastoral counselor.

In case that's not confusing enough, we'd like to mention psychoanalysts, mainly because they are the image that the media (and Oscar) hangs on to for its icon of psychiatry. Psychoanalysis is a very specific type of psychotherapy where the patient lies on a couch, facing away from the doctor, and talks about whatever comes to mind, a process known as free association. Therapy is conducted for three to five sessions a week and takes several years.

Psychoanalysis is the origin of all modern psychotherapies that base technique on the importance of unconscious thought, feelings, and intentions. The unique aspects of psychoanalysis include the frequency of the sessions, the importance of childhood experiences, and the focus on the patient's relationship with the psychoanalyst as a mirror of past relationships, a process called *transference.* The goals of psychoanalysis are an in-depth understanding of the unconscious experience and a greater flexibility in self experience that enables the patient to make more adaptive choices. Psychoanalysis is used both to treat mental illness—often anxiety, depression, and personality disorders—and for personal growth and awareness. Most analytic patients also take medications to address specific symptoms.

Psychoanalytic training typically takes five, or more, years and is done part time while the trainee works. It includes a personal psychoanalysis for the therapist. Traditionally, psychoanalysts have been psychiatrists, but that is no longer the case. Although the analytic couch is the image we often think of in connection with psychiatry, very few psychiatrists practice this form of treatment, and very few patients are treated with it. We mentioned the image of a bearded psychiatrist who smokes a cigar and sits behind the couch, but this is a caricature—we don't actually know of any doctors who still smoke while they see patients!

How does all this relate to our fictional patients?

Oscar Ford stayed in the Emergency Department (ED) for many hours. He spoke with the emergency room physician, a social worker, and then with a psychiatrist. Based on his history and mental status exam, it was determined that he was suffering from major depression and would benefit from ongoing psychiatric care, but this could be done on an outpatient basis, and the decision was made to release him. Oscar was given recommendations for follow-up, told that medications might be helpful, and discharged back to jail.

Melissa Adams called her personal physician to get the name of a psychiatrist and made an appointment within the week. When she called her insurance company to verify her benefits, she learned that the psychiatrist was not in her insurance company's network of providers. She trusted her personal physician's recommendation and decided to keep the appointment anyway, even though it would cost her more than it would to see a psychiatrist within her network. Melissa ultimately decided she didn't want an official record of her decision to get psychiatric treatment—she was afraid it might make it hard for her to get insurance later, so she decided to pay for her care out-of-pocket.

When Oscar Ford arrived at jail, he was taken to the booking officer. The arresting officer took off the handcuffs while the booking officer typed his information into a computer terminal. Oscar gave his name, date of birth, address, and then answered a series of questions about his medical history and about his recent drug and alcohol use. These included questions such as, Do you have heart disease, hypertension, diabetes, cancer or AIDS? Are you on any medications? Do you have any mental disorders and are you on any psychiatric medication? Are you suicidal? Finally, the officer made note of anything unusual about Oscar that might suggest he could be having a serious medical or mental health problem: obvious bleeding or broken bones, trouble breathing, confusion, emotional distress, or unusual or bizarre behavior. Once the screen was complete, Oscar was referred to an intake nurse for a more in-depth evaluation of any question to which he had answered "yes."

Oscar Ford told the intake nurse he had just been diagnosed with depression. He also told her that he'd had "a bit" to drink that evening. He denied any history of serious alcohol withdrawal problems. The nurse noted that he looked sad and withdrawn, and she asked him about a history of suicide attempts and if he had any present thoughts of harming himself. Oscar was not quite as irritable as he had been early in the evening when he'd been intoxicated, but he was annoyed by how many people had asked the same question over and over.

"Can't you just read my chart?" He snapped at the nurse. "I've been answering the same questions all night!"

She told him she could not. The Emergency Department psychiatrist had sent a brief note with treatment recommendations, but not a detailed history.

Oscar said no to both questions: he'd never tried to commit suicide, and he wasn't thinking about it now. The nurse noted that the ED psychiatrist had recommended medication for depression, and she filled out a referral form for the jail psychology department. She told the correctional officer on duty that Oscar was cleared for housing in the general population of the jail and that he did not require suicide observation. She told Oscar she would refer him to the psychiatrist.

Oscar saw the court commissioner and bail was set. Unfortunately, legal fees related to his divorce and custody battle had devoured his savings, and he couldn't make bail. A year ago, he'd been financially comfortable; now he was facing bankruptcy. He was held in jail pending trial. The jail psychologist logged in the psychiatric referral and then gave it to the clinic secretary, who scheduled Oscar for the next available psychiatry clinic.

Oscar saw a forensic psychiatrist. The doctor he saw had completed all the training that every psychiatrist does, as well as fellowship training in the subspecialty of forensic psychiatry. The term *forensic* comes from the Latin word *forum,* meaning "an open space," and refers to the law, because in ancient Rome, that's where legal matters were debated—in a public open space. Forensic psychiatrists have training in civil and criminal mental health issues. They testify as expert witnesses in many types of cases: criminal, insanity defenses, juvenile hearings, child custody and visitation, malpractice, and other cases. A forensic psychiatrist may have a private forensic practice or may work for a court system as an independent court-appointed expert.

In addition to providing consultation services for court cases, forensic psychiatrists also provide care to mentally ill people in secure settings. If a criminal defendant is too mentally ill to participate in a trial, he is confined to a psychiatric hospital for treatment, and a forensic psychiatrist will treat him there. If a defendant is found to be legally "insane," he will also be cared for by a forensic psychiatrist. Forensic psychiatrists have experience working in secure settings like state hospitals and correctional facilities, including jails and prisons. They are used to working with mentally ill people who are dangerous because of their illness or personality problems.

Oscar Ford hadn't done anything that carried a lengthy jail term, and legal sanity was never an issue in his case. The forensic psychiatrist saw him for treatment, explained that he had an illness called major depression, then started him on a medication. Oscar went off to his cell to await trial.

Oscar finally got out of jail when his sister returned from vacation and posted bail. The kind judge who heard his case ordered him to treatment as a condition of his probation. Probation agreements don't usually state which type of mental health professional a defendant should see, how often he should go, or what kind of psychiatric care he should get. Oscar had to figure all this out on his own.

He wanted to schedule an appointment, but he was confused. Should he see his internist for medications and recommendations? Should he see a psychotherapist for talk therapy? Should he see a psychiatrist, and if so, would the psychiatrist just prescribe medications and send him to another professional for psychotherapy, or would the psychiatrist see him for both components of treatment? The answers to these questions would depend on many things, including what Oscar could afford and what resources were available. Once he figured out his treatment options, he could make a decision based on the availability of care, his own resources, and his personal preference. Melissa Adams could afford the best of care, and she just assumed that the psychiatrist she was going to would see her for weekly therapy appointments.

Oscar decided to see a psychiatrist, but often mental illnesses, especially depression and anxiety, are treated by primary care doctors—family doctors, internists, or even gynecologists—not by psychiatrists. While there are always exceptions, here are some reasons a patient should see a psychiatrist and not a primary care doctor:

- Sometimes a patient's distress is overwhelming. The patient may repeatedly call her family doctor and worry a great deal about symptoms and medications. If the doctor is getting anxious about managing the patient and feels the case is becoming a burden for him, the patient should see a psychiatrist. Psychiatrists are better at dealing with distressed patients.
- Any patient with the new onset of a psychotic illness should initially be stabilized by a psychiatrist. A *psychotic* disorder is one in which the patient has hallucinations or delusions or both. Hallucinations mean that someone sees, hears, feels, or smells things that aren't there. Delusions are a fixed belief in something that isn't real. For example, a paranoid delusion might entail the belief that the government is watching the patient with special cameras. If this is truly happening, then it's not a delusion! Psychosis is frequently seen in schizophrenia and bipolar disorder but can also be seen with major depression, delirium, drug intoxication, and a host of other nonpsychiatric illnesses, such as severe thyroid disease or brain disorders. Primary care doctors don't typically

treat psychotic illnesses, and it just makes sense to have someone with expertise stabilize the patient.

• For major depression, a conservative recommendation is that a primary care doctor should refer to a psychiatrist after the patient fails one trial of antidepressant medication given at a therapeutic dose for long enough.

• All patients with bipolar disorder need a psychiatrist to stabilize them and to manage acute episodes. "Stability" is a relative term in psychiatry, but it generally means the patient is no longer behaving in a disorganized manner or having extremely distressing symptoms. If someone has been stable on lithium for the past eight years, he doesn't necessarily need a psychiatrist to prescribe it, but he may want one. If the patient has had even one manic episode, then prescribing antidepressants can be very risky, and a referral to a psychiatrist should be considered.

• Any patient with a recent serious suicide attempt or recent psychiatric hospitalization should be stabilized by a psychiatrist.

• Any patient with any psychiatric disorder that is compromising his ability to function, who does not improve after two to three months of treatment, should be referred for psychiatric care; for example, obsessive-compulsive disorder or panic disorder that is not getting better is best treated by a specialist.

• Primary care doctors should treat psychiatric disorders only if they are comfortable doing so. Some are; some aren't.

• A psychiatric disorder that puts anyone's life at risk is usually more than a primary care doctor wants to, or should, treat.

• Any patient being treated by a primary care doctor for a psychiatric illness should be asked if he wants to see a psychotherapist (a psychiatrist, psychologist, social worker, or nurse therapist). The patient may say that the pills have cured his depression and he doesn't need to talk, but psychotherapy is often helpful, and the gentle *offer* of a psychotherapy referral should be made early.

Oscar's best friend knew a psychiatrist, but the psychiatrist was not in his health insurance network, so he explained some of Oscar's options. Oscar was living paycheck to paycheck at this point and decided he couldn't afford to see anyone outside his network because he'd have a higher co-pay. He called the insurance company, got a list of doctors in his network, and started making phone calls. He became frustrated after finding that many of the doctors on the list had moved, retired, died, or were no longer taking patients. Some could not see him for three months. He called about a dozen or so numbers before he found a psychiatrist who was able to see him soon.

The doctor Oscar saw was in a group practice with two other psychiatrists, a psychologist, and seven social workers. The psychiatrist asked him many of the same questions he'd been asked in the ED and in jail. By this point, Oscar was feeling much better, and the psychiatrist refilled the medication that Oscar had started taking in jail, then referred him to one of the social workers for psychotherapy.

He was to return to the doctor in a month, and if his depression remained under control, he'd be seen every few months as long as he continued on medication. The doctor recommended that Oscar remain on the antidepressant for one year.

Melissa saw only a psychiatrist for her care, while Oscar had a treatment team consisting of a psychiatrist and a social worker. The type of care Oscar received is called *split treatment*. There are pros and cons of dividing psychiatric treatment versus having a single psychiatrist provide all the care.

Medications can be prescribed by a psychiatrist, any other medical doctor, a physician's assistant, or a nurse practitioner. In Louisiana and New Mexico, psychologists are now permitted to prescribe certain psychiatric medications if they've completed special courses and obtained a specific amount of supervision. Medication management focuses on an assessment of symptoms—such as mood, sleep, appetite, hallucinations, delusions, and anxiety-related problems—and issues related to prescribing medications. Many medications require monitoring of blood tests and electrocardiograms (EKGs) as well as consideration of what other medications the patient is taking. These visits are usually much shorter than psychotherapy sessions.

In many settings, split treatment is the rule. Community mental health centers cater to patients who have publicly funded insurance, such as Medicaid, or no resources at all. They also care for patients with chronic and severe mental illnesses. Neither Melissa nor Oscar fell into this category. In community clinics, social workers or nurse therapists see patients for psychotherapy, and the psychiatrist sees patients to make a diagnosis, to assess symptoms, and to prescribe and monitor medications. If all is going well, the patient is usually seen by a psychiatrist every one to three months (a ninety-day review is mandated by our state's regulations). If the patient is having symptoms or side effects, he is seen more often. Both the therapists and the psychiatrists use the same medical chart, and in clinics, the communication among the treatment team is usually good. In private practice, the patient may see a psychiatrist at one office and a psychotherapist at another, and communication between the two will vary, or it may not occur at all. Oscar's psychiatrist and social worker worked in the same office and were able to communicate easily.

There aren't enough psychiatrists for everyone everywhere to see one for psychotherapy. Some psychiatrists don't like seeing patients for psychotherapy. They may prefer the medical aspects of evaluating and treating illnesses. With such a strong emphasis on the biological aspects of psychiatric disorders, many residency training programs have de-emphasized the teaching of psychotherapy. Finally, insurance companies often reimburse psychiatrists better if they see more patients for less time, which discourages psychiatrists from seeing patients for longer psychotherapy appointments. Many believe that it is more cost effective to have psychiatrists prescribe medications and social workers do psychotherapy, but it's not clear that this is always true.

Patients in split therapy are often helped by their nonphysician psychotherapists and get good symptom relief from medications prescribed by a doctor who may see them for only fifteen minutes per month or per quarter, and they are pleased with their care and have good outcomes.

Still, in some circumstances, better care comes from having one practitioner manage both therapy and medications. Here are some reasons patients might want to see psychiatrists for both:

- A psychiatrist who does psychotherapy really gets to know the patients—they aren't just a compilation of symptoms. Psychiatric symptoms are often very similar to normal reactions, and a psychiatrist who knows a patient well can get a much better feel for when a symptom is a symptom and not just a reaction to circumstances.

• Some patients are prone to dividing their treatment team into a good guy and a bad guy. With these patients, the people treating them may end up taking sides, and the noise of the relationships overwhelms the task of helping the patient to get better. Patients who have certain types of personality disorders are more likely to have this situation and miss out on good therapeutic care as a result.

• Nonphysician therapists may overlook or explain away episodes of major mental illness such that the patient never gets an appropriate referral for medications. A patient may have a perfectly good, caring relationship with a therapist and feel comforted and understood but not get cured because a diagnosis is missed. It is normal for people to be upset during a divorce, and Oscar's distress could have been attributed to his circumstances. The severity and duration of his symptoms, however, indicated that he was suffering from major depression.

• One-stop shopping is more convenient.

• Seeing a psychiatrist for both medications and therapy is typically cheaper than seeing both a psychologist (for psychotherapy) and a psychiatrist (for medications) since many Ph.D.-level psychologists charge as much as psychiatrists.

We don't believe that *every* psychiatric patient is best served, however, by seeing only a psychiatrist, and split treatment is sometimes the best treatment. Patients with severe and persistent mental illnesses, who are disabled by their disease, often require coordinated care between agencies, and the time that would otherwise be allotted for psychotherapy is used to arrange for these services. These patients may need day programs, vocational training, housing, help obtaining government benefits and health insurance, transportation to appointments, and even outreach to their homes to make sure they are getting and taking their medications. Social workers and case managers do a better job than psychiatrists of helping patients obtain these resources, because they do this on a regular basis. For these patients, talk therapy in the traditional sense may be a limited part of care, and what makes the biggest difference in their lives is help in accessing services and treatment.

Split treatment, particularly in a clinic setting, may be the most practical care in other situations as well:

- Patients with chronic mental illnesses may need help in coordinating their care. Mental health professionals may need to work with home care providers, supported employment programs, and psychosocial rehabilitation centers. Social workers know more than psychiatrists about program coordination.
- It may be cheaper for a clinic to pay a social worker than a psychiatrist (or a doctoral-level psychologist).
- Split therapy works best if the psychotherapist is readily available for consultation. In a clinic setting, this communication occurs easily, and the patient has a single chart that both professionals share.

Some psychiatrists are lousy psychotherapists. Some psychiatrists have no interest in doing psychotherapy, and some patients have no interest in being seen for psychotherapy. Many mental health practices are not set up for the psychiatrist to do psychotherapy, often because insurance companies have fee-reimbursement structures that make it financially impractical for the most trained, and therefore most expensive, mental health professional to spend as much time with patients as psychotherapy requires.

Medications are often helpful even when they are prescribed by a psychiatrist with the social skills of an iguana. Psychotherapy, however, requires some degree of connection, some sense that the therapist can empathize. Without this, it simply doesn't work as a treatment modality. There's not a therapist out there who is the perfect therapist for everyone, and some people don't like even the "best" psychotherapists.

In many settings, the only option is for patients to have treatment split, and it doesn't mean that the patient is getting substandard care. What if a patient begins psychotherapy with a psychologist or social worker and finds this very helpful but still needs medications? Should she jump ship to see a psychiatrist for psychotherapy? Probably not, but it is best if the patient sees a psychiatrist who has a working relationship with her therapist.

Oscar Ford did well in his treatment. The medication helped his mood, his sleep, and his appetite. He stopped being so withdrawn, stopped crying every night, and stopped drinking heavily. He was a man with concerns aside from a simple biological depression: he was grieving the dissolution of his marriage, he was lonely, he was behaving badly, and he was abusing alcohol. He received education about his medicine and his illness. He found some relief in talking about his problems and was able to take a more in-depth look at the events and relationships in his past that influenced how he handled stress and related to others in the present.

Melissa Adams saw a psychiatrist for a psychiatric evaluation. She talked a lot about the struggles she had watched her father go through with major depression, and in fact, several other family members had suffered with the illness, including an uncle who committed suicide. She talked about the stress of balancing a career and a family, and she relayed to the psychiatrist that while she had a terrific professional reputation, she felt like a fake who didn't deserve to be so well thought of. She'd had trouble getting along with one of the doctors in her group, and her youngest son was not doing well in school. Melissa had been healthy, except for an ankle injury she'd sustained while rock climbing in her twenties; she'd required several surgeries to reconstruct the joint, and she still sometimes took ibuprofen, an over-the-counter pain medication. Recently she put on some weight, and her sex drive was completely gone.

Melissa's psychiatrist ordered blood tests, including thyroid function tests because depression can be a symptom of hypothyroidism. She started Melissa on a medication and told her to return in one week. The psychiatrist felt Melissa would benefit from both psychotherapy and medication.

Oscar saw a psychiatrist five times over the course of a year. He had a good response to the medication, and his depression resolved. He completed the terms of his probation and did not continue to drink excessively. In psychotherapy with a social worker, Oscar came to understand some important things about his contribution to a failed marriage, and he found the support he needed to get through a very difficult time in his life. Once his behavior improved, his wife did not hesitate to let him see the children, and a joint custody arrangement was finalized.

Melissa did not respond to the first medication she tried. She began a second medication and had intolerable side effects. The third medication helped, but ultimately she needed to be on two medications before her depression fully lifted. She saw the psychiatrist weekly for a while, but once her depression was better, she found it difficult to make time for the sessions, and she didn't feel a need for weekly therapy sessions. She continued with therapy but only went once every six weeks. Because it had been so difficult to treat her depression, Melissa did not want to stop the medications after a year, and she continued on them for quite some time.

Chapter 2

Josh:
A Walk through the System

JOSH TAYLOR was the best player on his high school soccer team, even though he suffered from asthma. He had always been a good student, was not bad on the guitar, and he didn't have any trouble making friends in the dorm when he went away to college. Josh was very tall, and his brown eyes sang from beneath a sweep of dark hair. His wry sense of humor kept people on their toes. He was a polite kid, but sometimes he seemed just a little bit shy.

In the spring semester of his sophomore year, Josh shut down. He stopped hanging out with his friends, and he hardly ever went to class. He even lost interest in 24, his favorite TV show. He slept a lot—even for a college student—and still, he was tired all the time. When he went home for spring break, his parents were shocked to see how thin he'd gotten. His doctor could find nothing physically wrong, and Josh told him that he was feeling pretty down and hopeless. Josh's doctor thought he was probably suffering from a psychiatric disorder and recommended an evaluation by a psychiatrist.

Like Oscar and Melissa, Josh is not a real person. Unlike Oscar and Melissa, Josh does not suffer from major depression, and his story has more twists. We've created Josh to illustrate how psychiatrists think about complicated patients in different treatment settings.

The purpose of a psychiatric evaluation depends, in part, on where it is conducted. In settings where the patient will be seen for ongoing treatment, the psychiatric evaluation is used to determine the nature of the problem, make a diagnosis, and formulate a treatment plan. The evaluation offers the psychiatrist a chance to gather the patient's history, and it gives the patient a chance to see if he's comfortable working with that psychiatrist. In a private practice setting, the evaluation is usually done by the treating psychiatrist. In a clinic, the evaluation may be done by one psychiatrist, and the patient may then be seen by another psychiatrist for treatment. On a hospital inpatient unit, several factors determine whether the evaluating psychiatrist will continue with the patient's treatment or a different doctor will take over the patient's care. For example, in teaching hospitals the patient may be evaluated by several doctors, and people admitted on weekends and off-hours may be seen by a covering psychiatrist.

In an Emergency Department, the purpose of a psychiatric evaluation is much different. The mental health professionals in the ED will not offer extended treatment. The doctor's goals are to determine whether the patient requires hospitalization, and if not, to provide referrals for outpatient resources. The focus in the ED is on safety and on the acute symptoms that brought the patient to attention, not on gathering a complete history or providing treatment beyond what is necessary for immediate stabilization.

When Josh mentioned that he had thought about suicide, his doctor initially told him to go to the ED for an evaluation.

"I'm not going to off myself," Josh said. "I think about it sometimes, but I'm not going to do it." He really did not want to go to the Emergency Department for a psychiatric evaluation.

"Do you promise you'll go to the ER if you think you might hurt yourself?" the doctor finally asked.

"Yes. I'm not going to kill myself," Josh repeated.

Josh's doctor was understandably worried, and he asked Josh's mother to come in from the waiting room and join them. Josh was 18, so he could have refused to allow his physician to talk with his mother, but he didn't. Josh's mother spoke with the doctor and agreed to watch Josh closely, and to get him to a psychiatrist as soon as possible.

The psychiatrist's office looked a little like Josh's dad's office at home. It was lit with lamps, and the overhead fluorescent lights remained off.

There was artwork on the walls, a small area rug, knickknacks here and there, some plants, and a lot of books on shelves, but no family photographs. Dr. Nathan Smith was a short man with a bit of a pot belly. He was in his early thirties and had sandy hair and a moustache. He sat at a desk, and Josh settled in across from him. In the corner were two comfortable-looking chairs, where they would sit during subsequent therapy sessions. For that first appointment, the psychiatrist took notes while they talked, but he often looked up and met Josh's eyes. Dr. Smith had a gentle manner and was a good listener.

The questions psychiatrists ask depend on their theoretical orientation. Some traditional psychoanalysts let the patient tell their own story and ask very few questions. Most psychiatrists do a structured interview to collect specific information. It's important to note that a psychiatric evaluation is not psychotherapy, and therapy sessions may be much less structured.

Dr. Smith began by asking Josh what was troubling him—what doctors call the chief complaint. He then asked when the problem started and what may have triggered it. Was there a precipitating event, such as a breakup or the death of someone close? Did the difficulties come on suddenly or gradually? What symptoms were present and how much were they interfering with Josh's life? This portion of the evaluation is called the history of present illness.

"I just don't feel like doing anything," Josh said.

"Nothing?" Dr. Smith asked.

"Not really. I keep saying I'm going to go to class, but then I wake up in the middle of the night and can't sleep. When I do fall back to sleep, I sleep through the alarm." Josh thought for a moment and added, "Sometimes I play video games."

"What do you like to play?" the doctor asked. He asked about specific video games for a number of reasons. For one thing, he wanted to form a rapport with Josh. He also wanted to get a sense of Josh and his life. Did he play war games or sports games? By himself, with friends, or online? How many hours a day? Josh played a soccer video game on Xbox, by himself, for about two or three hours a day.

Psychiatrists have different interview styles. Dr. Smith listened while Josh talked about how difficult things had been that semester. He then asked Josh if they could talk about his past and come back to the current problem later. This question served as a transition, and by asking for permission, Dr. Smith gave Josh some control over the process. The doctor liked to get a sense of the patient and how his life had transpired before he heard much about the illness.

Dr. Smith asked questions about his family: Who was in it? What were their occupations? Were they healthy? What were their personalities like, and what kind of relationship did Josh have with them?

His father had died when he was a toddler, so when Josh talked about his parents, he meant his mother and stepfather. Josh was very close to his stepsister, Janine. They talked on Facebook almost every day. He got along "okay" with his stepfather. Stan was a patent attorney, and he'd married Josh's mom when Josh was four. He had a temper.

Dr. Smith asked about any history of psychiatric illness in family members, specifically blood relatives, and he asked the question in several different ways because genetics are so important in psychiatry.

"My mother has bipolar disorder," Josh said. "She takes Depakote."

"Has she been hospitalized?"

"I think so. Before I was born. And she was depressed for a while right after I was born." Josh looked around the office for a moment, then continued. "She's moody a lot, and when Stan gets annoyed with her, he says she's going through menopause."

Josh did not know of any other family history of psychiatric illness.

"Has anyone in your family died of suicide?"

"No," Josh replied.

Once Dr. Smith learned about the family, he asked Josh about his personal history. Did he have any problems in childhood with his health, behavior, or development? Dr. Smith also asked Josh about his education, work history, encounters with the law, and romantic relationships. He asked about drug and alcohol use, medical and surgical history, a list of current medications, and drug allergies.

Dr. Smith learned that Josh had trouble sitting still in school as a young child, and that several teachers suggested he might have problems with attention and hyperactivity, but Josh's mother did not want him to take medications. In second grade, she moved him to a school with smaller classes, and after that, he did very well academically. Josh had always loved sports, and he was very athletic and coordinated. It didn't hurt that he was six feet tall by tenth grade.

Josh liked college, at least at first. He partied a bit too much the first semester and was surprised at how difficult his schoolwork was. He had a new girlfriend, and at first, he'd thought he was in love, but now he wasn't so sure. He sheepishly admitted that he smoked pot and drank beer on weekends, and he had tried cocaine once but had no interest in doing it again. He'd last drank alcohol and smoked marijuana over the past weekend.

Josh had fairly severe asthma, and he'd been to the Emergency Department a couple of times a year as a child for acute episodes of bronchospasm. He'd been admitted to the hospital twice and had been on steroids, but he had never required a respirator. Josh talked about his asthma as "no big deal," but he still took medications for it and carried an inhaler with him. His last treatment in the ED for an asthma attack was in September, shortly after he'd started college.

Josh had his tonsils and adenoids out when he was five. His nose was broken when he was hit with a football, and he was pleased to report that he'd played out the game anyway, and they had won. He was allergic to sulfa drugs—they gave him a rash—and pollen.

By this point in an interview, Dr. Smith had some idea of who his patient was as a person, who was important in his life, and some of the crucial events that had transpired. Finally, he asked about past psychiatric encounters. What's important? Past diagnoses, hospitalizations, episodes of suicidality and violence, and what treatments have been tried. He wanted to know the responses to every treatment: Were the outcomes good or bad or something in between? If medications have been used, then he'd ask about each medication, the maximum dose that was taken, the response and any side effects, and why the medication was stopped. Dr. Smith wanted to know if Josh had ever seen a counselor or therapist, and if his pediatrician or primary care doctor had ever prescribed medicines for behavioral or emotional problems, like depression or anxiety.

Josh had never seen a mental health professional before, but in high school he'd had a pretty rough period after a girlfriend broke up with him, and he felt now a bit like he'd felt back then. He had not been as depressed during that episode, but his grades did drop for a marking period. Josh had never had any symptoms of mania, a condition in which mood, energy, and activity are elevated rather than depressed.

The final part of the psychiatric evaluation is called the mental status exam. This is the psychiatrist's version of a physical exam, only it's not physical. The doctor assesses and describes the patient, much as a novelist might write a character analysis, but in a formulaic way.

Dr. Smith observed and recorded anything remarkable about Josh's appearance. Josh was a neatly groomed and casually dressed young man in jeans, a T-shirt, and flip flops. He was quite slim, and his jeans were loose. His hair was long—so long that he had to continually brush his bangs from his eyes to see. Josh was cooperative with the interview, but he rarely made eye contact with his new doctor.

Dr. Smith looked for any abnormal movements, such as tics or an abnormal gait, which could be a sign of a neurological problem, and Josh had none. He considered Josh's speech, and noted whether it was clear and coherent and normal in rate and volume. Dr. Smith asked Josh about his mood, his energy, and his participation in his usual activities. He asked specific questions about feelings of hopelessness, death wishes, or suicidal thoughts. Josh mentioned that his senses felt dulled—colors didn't seem as bright, and food didn't taste as good. He didn't care about sex anymore, which was striking.

Dr. Smith asked if Josh was having any unusual perceptions. Did he hear voices or see things that were not there? False perceptions are called hallucinations. How was his assessment of reality? Was he suffering from any delusions? Delusions are fixed false beliefs, and are often paranoid in nature.

Josh looked offended. "I'm not crazy!"

Dr. Smith smiled. "I don't think you're crazy, but I'm a psychiatrist, so I ask everyone these questions. Please don't be offended."

Dr. Smith asked about obsessions, compulsions, and phobias. Some psychiatrists do this as part of the history, while others do it during the mental status exam.

Finally, Dr. Smith assessed Josh's cognitive state. He asked questions about orientation, for example, asking Josh where he was and what the date was. If there is any concern about cognition, Dr. Smith might administer a test called the Mini-Mental Status Exam (MMSE) to get a quick and objective measure of how well the patient is oriented and whether attention, recall, memory, and concentration are intact. Some psychiatrists ask patients to interpret proverbs, such as "People who live in glass houses shouldn't throw stones." While such a question may seem obscure during the course of an interview, it can help the psychiatrist gain some insight into the patient's ability to think abstractly. Finally, the psychiatrist makes an estimate of the patient's intelligence, insight, and judgment. In Josh's case, Dr. Smith didn't see any need to ask any of these questions. As Josh talked about his life, it was obvious that his brain was working fine. Josh easily recalled dates and details, knew what medications he was on, and could talk about current events, especially those related to sports and music. Dr. Smith did not need to ask specific questions or do any testing because he had gotten the same information in more subtle ways. Josh was obviously of average or above average intelligence, and his memory was intact.

A mental status exam sounds clinical because it is. It's a psychiatrist's attempt to describe a patient's mental functioning as a snapshot in time. We do our best to infer someone's internal experiences from what we observe and what they report. It's meant to be a description of these observations, one that we try not to cloud with our own judgments or feelings.

After the mental status exam, any relevant laboratory or radiologic tests are noted. Josh's primary care doctor had checked his blood count, because anemia can cause fatigue, and his thyroid, because hypothyroidism can cause symptoms of depression and fatigue. A routine blood chemistry panel revealed that his liver and kidneys were all functioning fine and that he did not have diabetes. A blood level was checked for his asthma medication, and it was fine. A drug screen was positive for cannabis.

After the data collection was completed, Dr. Smith wrote a formal diagnostic impression. He listed the important findings and included his thoughts about the contributing or complicating factors, and the pros and cons of different treatments. He made two diagnoses and listed other diagnoses to be ruled out or considered. The written psychiatric evaluation would not be given to Josh, though a copy might be sent to Josh's primary care doctor if Josh was comfortable with this.

Dr. Smith believed Josh had major depression, moderate to severe in intensity, possibly recurrent, without any psychotic phenomena (meaning Josh was not having hallucinations or delusions). Josh also met criteria for a diagnosis of cannabis abuse. The family history of bipolar disorder was noted, and Dr. Smith included "Rule out bipolar disorder, depressed" in the differential diagnosis, but since Josh had never had a manic episode, he could not be diagnosed with bipolar disorder. It was something to be aware of because sometimes young people develop depression first, then later have an episode of mania, and Josh did have a family history. The doctor noted that Josh had asthma, listed current stressors, and assessed Josh's overall level of functioning, which was quite impaired.

Dr. Smith then outlined a course of treatment, which included starting a medication and psychotherapy. He told Josh that alcohol and marijuana might be contributing to his problems and suggested that Josh might want to avoid them. Josh was given a prescription for an antidepressant, and Dr. Smith told him some of the more common side effects. He warned Josh that antidepressants could cause suicidal thoughts in a small percentage of young people and could trigger a manic episode. He was especially concerned about this because Josh's mother had bipolar disorder. He educated Josh about the symptoms of mania and told him to call if he experienced any of these symptoms.

"People can hear voices or believe they have special powers when they are manic," Dr. Smith warned.

He wished that Josh had brought his mother with him. That way, he could obtain a more complete family history and he could tell her what to watch for as Josh started the medication.

The diagnostic interview provides a great deal of information, but it may not include all the information that is needed. That's why psychiatrists often want to get information from collateral sources such as a spouse, parents, or adult children. The word *collateral* in this sense just means "from people other than the patient." Occasionally, psychiatrists need to rely on information from a neighbor or an employer when there is no family and the person has been acting strangely at work or in the neighborhood. The amount of effort used to collect this information is directly proportional to the perceived risk of coming to a wrong conclusion. For example, it is common to obtain collateral information in an Emergency Department, where there are often concerns about dangerousness, suicidality, or unusual behavior. This is especially important when an emergency petition for an involuntary evaluation has been filed by the police or a court.

In an inpatient psychiatric setting, there is often a need for collateral information. The situation is not as urgent as in an emergency room, because there is more time to get to know patients and to observe their symptoms and behaviors. Nonetheless, it is common to have a family meeting during a hospital stay. This gives us an opportunity to observe interactions with the family, obtain additional information, discuss the appropriateness of the discharge timing, and plan aftercare support. We talk more about emergency petitions and hospitalizations as we go along.

In an outpatient setting, collateral information is usually not as critical, though it may be helpful when people have illnesses that alter their judgment, such as addictions or bipolar disorder. There is a greater chance with these disorders that the patient will leave out important information. Sometimes people are not aware that they should report certain behaviors, other times they are embarrassed about their symptoms, and sometimes they simply wish to withhold important information.

Josh was a good informant. He was able to report his symptoms and talk about his life. His mother was not absolutely necessary for the treatment to continue, but if Josh didn't mind, Dr. Smith thought it might be helpful to meet her once to get more history and to include her in the discussions about the risks and benefits of medication.

When Josh told his parents he'd been diagnosed with major depression, his mother said she'd been told her bipolar disorder was due to a chemical imbalance, and she asked whether he also had one.

"Dr. Smith didn't actually say that," Josh said. "He said mood disorders are genetic. He said the medicine for the depression could unmask bipolar disorder, and I could have that and just not know it yet."

"Ask him if you have a chemical imbalance," Josh's mother said.

Chemical imbalance is a term with imprecise meaning, one that may absolve patients and their families of unwarranted guilt. Josh's parents might wonder, for example, if poor parenting caused his problems, or if he had lousy coping skills. One event in Josh's childhood is associated with an increased risk for depression: the death of a parent before age 11. Still, this doesn't answer the question of whether he has a chemical imbalance.

Saying that a psychiatric disorder is caused by a chemical imbalance, although an imperfect explanation, sometimes makes psychiatric disorders more palatable to patients and less stigmatizing. The term gives some credence to the practice of treating these disorders with medication. But there is no psychiatric disorder for which we know for certain which chemicals are "imbalanced," if any.

We have reasons for believing that psychiatric disorders must certainly be mediated by biological factors. For one thing, psychiatric illnesses run in families, even when family members are separated at birth. Research has shown that genetic links, and even specific genes, may be associated with different disorders. Many studies have shown that the biological features of groups of people with illnesses are different from those same features in groups of people without those illnesses. What we don't have, yet, is a specific reliable test for a certain genotype or enzyme level, or a brain scan finding that indicates that a specific person has a specific disease. Someone who goes to the doctor because of increased thirst and urination and has a lab test done that shows a markedly elevated blood sugar level most certainly has diabetes. With rare exceptions (e.g., Huntington's disease, Jacob-Creutzfelt dementia), there's nothing like this in psychiatry—no blood test, no x-ray, no CT scan that yields a definitive diagnosis. In psychiatry, blood tests are ordered to rule out medical conditions that masquerade as psychiatric illness, such as thyroid conditions or high ammonia levels, or to monitor medication levels and be certain the medications are not damaging the patient's organs.

We know that the medications used to treat mental illnesses alter the levels of certain neurotransmitters. The antidepressant Prozac increases levels of serotonin in the brain. We don't know for sure that depression is caused by low levels of serotonin, or that raising these levels is the mechanism that helps to alleviate the symptoms, but many lines of evidence suggest such a connection. In simpler terms, we presume there is a "chemical imbalance," but it remains uncertain as to what that imbalance actually is. Serotonin may be just one step in the final common pathway, along with many other steps, that contribute to the syndrome of depression. Simply said, we don't know the exact biological nature of what is wrong when someone has a mental illness; nor do we know for certain the exact mechanism by which medications or other treatments work.

For now, it is our assumption that Josh suffers from some type of chemical imbalance and that he might well benefit from taking a medication. We do know that people who have a parent with bipolar disorder are more likely to get bipolar disorder than people without those genes. And they are more likely to get bipolar disorder than random people in the population, even if they were given up for adoption at birth and raised by parents who do not have mental illness. Psychiatric disorders are not simply the result of learned behaviors or coping styles.

Josh met criteria for a psychiatric disorder called major depression, but what does that mean? What are these criteria? How do they get determined? Because psychiatrists deal with conditions and syndromes that can be a little hard to define, we use a manual that lists all psychiatric diagnoses and the symptoms that must be present to make any specific diagnosis. This allows us to be sure that a physician in one state or country who uses the term *panic disorder* is referring to the same exact condition that another clinician is referring to when using the same term. The name of this manual is the *Diagnostic and Statistical Manual*, or DSM. The most current edition is the DSM-IV-TR, which means it is the fourth edition with a text revision. The fifth edition is being worked on now and will be published in 2013.

The first classification of psychiatric disorders came out in 1917. It was called the "Statistical Manual for the Use of Institutions for the Insane," and it was a list of twenty-two rudimentary diagnoses. The military later adapted it for World War II, and the American Psychiatric Association further revised it into the first DSM in 1952. It has come to be known as the bible of psychiatry.

In practice, the diagnostic criteria have become a sort of Chinese menu—five symptoms from column A, two from column B, must have C and D, and voilà, you've got Diagnosis X. This rigid and formalized manner of establishing a psychiatric diagnosis has been a boon to research because we do not mix diagnostic apples and oranges.

Sure, it would be nice if we could run a definitive test and say, "Yes, the

Depression Factor is present in your blood; you've got major depression, single episode, and the level is seventy-five, so it's 'moderate.'" Or maybe, "The left side of the amygdala is enlarged; therefore it's panic disorder." Or, "The frontal region has increased metabolism when you spin around, so you've got paranoid schizophrenia." But it doesn't work that way (not now), and we don't have any definitive tests, other than a clinical evaluation. Which means we talk, we observe, and sometimes we get collateral information from family members or friends.

This is what the DSM criteria for major depression look like:

Diagnosis of Major Depressive Disorder, Single Episode
(Summarized from the *Diagnostic and
Statistical Manual of Mental Disorders*, fourth edition)

A. The person experiences a single major depressive episode.

1. For a major depressive episode a person must have experienced at least five of the nine symptoms below for the same two weeks or more, for most of the time almost every day; and this is a change from his/her prior level of functioning. One of the symptoms must be either (a) depressed mood, or (b) loss of interest.

a. Depressed mood. For children and adolescents, this may be irritable mood.

b. A significantly reduced level of interest or pleasure in most or all activities.

c. A considerable loss or gain of weight (e.g., 5 percent or more change of weight in a month when not dieting). This may also be an increase or decrease in appetite. For children, they may not gain an expected amount of weight.

d. Difficulty falling or staying asleep (insomnia), or sleeping more than usual (hypersomnia).

e. Behavior that is agitated or slowed down. Others should be able to observe this.

f. Feeling fatigued or having diminished energy.

g. Thoughts of worthlessness or extreme guilt (not about being ill).

h. Ability to think, concentrate, or make decisions is reduced.

i. Frequent thoughts of death or suicide (with or without a specific plan), or attempt of suicide.

2. The person's symptoms do not indicate a mixed episode.

3. The person's symptoms are a cause of great distress or difficulty in functioning at home, work, or other important areas.

4. The person's symptoms are not caused by substance use (e.g., alcohol, drugs, medication) or a medical disorder.

5. The person's symptoms are not due to normal grief or bereavement over the death of a loved one, they continue for more than two months, or they include great difficulty in functioning, frequent thoughts of worthlessness, thoughts of suicide, symptoms that are psychotic, or behavior that is slowed down (psychomotor retardation).

B. Another disorder does not better explain the major depressive episode.

C. The person has never had a manic, mixed, or a hypomanic episode (unless an episode was due to a medical disorder or use of a substance).

Possible specifiers to describe the episode:
Severity: mild, moderate, severe without psychotic features
Severe With Psychotic Features
In Partial/Full Remission
With Catatonic Features
With Melancholic Features
With Atypical Features
With Postpartum Onset

Josh started taking a low dose of sertraline, the generic form of Zoloft, and three days later, he was no longer depressed, but he seemed *too* well, too fast. He slept very little, and he talked very quickly. He had a lot of ideas and plans. His mother phoned Dr. Smith, and he told her to stop the sertraline. The antidepressant had induced an episode of mania in Josh. It was likely, Dr. Smith said, that Josh had bipolar disorder, and it would be safer for him to take a mood stabilizer. The doctor thought this because of Josh's genetic predisposition to bipolar disorder as well as the

antidepressant-induced episode of mania. If a mania is caused by a medication, it is not completely clear that the patient has bipolar disorder, but
in Josh's case, Zoloft was obviously not the right medication for him. He
saw Dr. Smith the next day and started a new medication.

Josh got better. He returned to college, and things went well. For a
while, anyway. He continued taking the mood stabilizer, and he saw a
doctor at school for psychotherapy sessions.

In November, the flu started going around. One cold Friday afternoon, Josh played a long pickup game of soccer. He felt a little sick, but
he figured it was just a cold. By the end of the game, his chest was tight,
and he used his inhaler. Still, he went to party with his friends after. They
met in a dorm room, where they had a few beers and smoked marijuana.
Some of the boys also smoked cigarettes, and the room got pretty smoky.
Soon, Josh was coughing and struggling to breathe. His wheezing was
audible across the room, and he had a fever. The inhaler didn't help at all.
A friend finally brought him to the emergency room.

Josh had the flu, but that wasn't his only problem. The flu, exercise in
the cold air, and inhaling smoke had all contributed to a serious asthma
attack. In the Emergency Department, Josh was started on intravenous
fluids and given nebulizer treatments for his asthma. Hours later, he continued to wheeze, and his oxygen saturation was still a little low. He was
given intravenous steroids and admitted to the hospital.

Josh stayed for two days until his breathing was clear and his fever had
broken. He went home with a prescription for prednisone, a steroid; instructions to taper the medication over a few days; and a clear message
not to smoke anything. Josh was warned that the steroids could induce
a manic episode, but he felt fine when he left the hospital. His parents
came to visit, and they wanted Josh to go home with them and rest for a
few days, but Josh insisted he felt fine and was worried about falling behind in his schoolwork.

Within a few days, Josh was manic again, even though he was still
taking a mood stabilizer. Steroids can cause mania in people who are predisposed to it, and sometimes even in people who aren't.

This time, Josh's mania was not subtle, and it came on very quickly. He
was up all night watching recorded episodes of 24, and soon he had the
sense that he and Jack Bauer, the main character, were somehow linked.

He heard voices and thought someone wanted to hurt him, then he charged with a knife at his roommate (who had fast reflexes and ducked). The campus police were called, and Josh was brought to the ED for a psychiatric evaluation.

The ED can be a chaotic place. That night, it was busy, and all around things were loud, stimulating, and not so pleasant smelling. An intoxicated man was sleeping on a stretcher while an intravenous line nourished him with a yellow fluid. A dirty homeless man with no shoes sat in the hallway. An agitated woman yelled at the doctor every time he walked past, "I gotta go home and get my kids!" All told, there was one doctor, two nurses, and seven psychiatric patients. Some sat quietly and looked a bit forlorn; one paced; and everyone required a fair amount of attention. The fluorescent lights didn't allow for any tranquility, and overhead announcements blared every few minutes over the din of distraught conversations and assorted cell phones ringing.

Josh was so wired that he barely noticed all the racket. Someone wanted his insurance information (he told her where to stick it); another person took his blood pressure and pulse; and a third wanted his blood.

The psychiatrist in the ED learned that Josh had bipolar disorder and had been stable on medication. He checked the level of this medication in Josh's blood, and the level was good. Josh had not skipped any doses. The steroids that Josh needed to treat his asthma had triggered an episode of mania, and he still needed them for a few more days.

"I'm not crazy!" Josh yelled. "They'll kill me up there! I know it."

"I'm not trying to hurt you," the doctor said. "In fact, I'm trying to help you."

"Liar! I am only interested in what's best for my country!"

He yelled something about Tony, and Josh's roommate told the psychiatrist that Tony was a character from *24*. The psychiatrist spoke to Josh's mother, to Dr. Smith, and to the doctor Josh was seeing at school. Josh was given a medication to help him calm down, but he threw it at the nurse. The ED staff was frightened; Josh was out of control; and when Josh pushed a cup of water out of the nurse's hand, a security guard held him down while the nurse injected a sedative the doctor had ordered. Josh continued to pace and yell, even when no one was in the room. He refused to sign in voluntarily.

When a second doctor came to examine him, Josh repeated that people were trying to kill him. He cursed at the doctor and didn't make much sense, so it was a very brief visit. This second doctor had not come to do a complete evaluation but to give a second opinion on the necessity of involuntary commitment. Two doctors must agree on this by law.

Both physicians agreed that Josh was suffering from a mental illness and that he was a danger to others because of it. There was no less restrictive place where Josh could get treatment and still remain safe, and they filled out paperwork to start the involuntary admission process. Josh was escorted to a locked psychiatric unit.

Involuntary psychiatric admission, also known as civil commitment, did not always exist in the United States. This is because people cared for those with mental illness at home or in private hospitals, if the patient came from a wealthy family. Public psychiatric hospitals were created in the 1840s through the efforts of the reformer Dorothea Dix. Psychiatric patients were admitted without any legal protections or due process. For example, in the nineteenth century, men could sign their wives into a psychiatric hospital without a hearing or any proof of mental illness, and the women could be held in the hospital indefinitely. Fortunately, that's not how commitment happens today.

The government allows people to be civilly committed for two reasons. First, the state has an obligation to protect the public. If someone's mental illness makes him dangerous to himself or others, he can be admitted involuntarily. This is known as the *police powers* basis for civil commitment. The *parens patriae* doctrine is the other reason for commitment. *Parens patriae* literally means "in the place of the parent." In other words, it is the government's responsibility to care for people who are unable to care for themselves.

Certain legal steps have to be followed to commit a patient to a hospital. The first step is to transport the patient to an emergency room for evaluation by a mental health professional. The police transported our fictional patient, Josh, to the hospital just as they did Oscar Ford in the last chapter. In some jurisdictions, this is known as an emergency petition process. An emergency petition is a legal document that allows the police to pick someone up and transport him to a psychiatric evaluation, even if he doesn't want to go. A psychiatrist or other mental health professional may fill out an emergency petition form. A law enforcement officer can fill one out if the officer observes evidence that the patient is dangerous. This happened with Josh—he was screaming and agitated when the police arrived. Any concerned citizen can go before a judge and request an emergency psychiatric evaluation on behalf of an ill person; however, the judge must approve the request and sign the form for it to be legally valid. In general, the patient must have been recently dangerous to himself or others to have an emergency evaluation carried out. After the patient arrives in the emergency room, he is evaluated by a mental health professional to determine if he needs to be admitted to the hospital or if he is safe to be discharged back into the community.

Josh was certified to the hospital so he could be involuntarily admitted for a brief period of observation. There is a statutory limit to the number of days a patient can be held for observation; for example, in Maryland this is ten days, although a seven-day extension can be requested. During this time, the inpatient psychiatrist determines if the patient is well enough to be discharged or if he requires a longer involuntary admission, as was the case for Josh.

If the patient needs to stay in the hospital, the psychiatrist begins formal civil commitment proceedings. Josh was given notice that a hearing would take place, and he received written information about his rights at the hearing, such as the right to representation and to cross-examine witnesses. The commitment hearing took place in a conference room in the hospital before an administrative law judge. In some states, a hearing officer makes the decision about commitment. Regardless, the judge or hearing officer is required to consider other, less restrictive means of treating the patient, such as outpatient care.

The judge's decision about commitment is based on each state's civil commitment law. The legal criteria for commitment are known as the commitment standard. Once, the commitment standard was extremely loose; to commit someone, the hospital had to show only that the patient was "in need of care." This changed in the 1970s, when the United States Supreme Court issued its landmark opinion in *Lessard v. Schmidt*. In *Lessard*, the Supreme Court said that the loss of liberty in civil commitment was serious enough to require hospitals to prove that the patient had a mental illness, and that as a result of the mental illness, he was a danger to himself or others. This standard, the dangerousness standard, has been criticized by many advocacy groups as being too stringent. A more lenient standard for commitment is the grave disability standard. In this case, the hospital needs only to prove that the patient is unable to care for himself or is at risk of serious harm due to self-neglect. Advocates favor this standard because it allows for the care of people with mental illness who also suffer from medical disease. For example, someone with active schizophrenia and diabetes who is unable to monitor his own blood sugar and medication could be committed to receive both psychiatric and medical care. Josh did not resist treatment for his asthma, but his psychiatric condition rendered him dangerous, and the fact that he had already threatened someone with a deadly weapon made his dangerousness clear.

The purpose of having a hearing and legal standards for commitment is to protect people from having their freedom taken away by mistake. Some patients are released at the civil commitment hearing, and the hospital must then discharge the patient. About 10 percent of patients who are taken to commitment hearings end up being released. Patients who are committed are allowed to appeal the decision, usually to a circuit court. They also have a right to a lay adviser or legal counsel at both the commitment hearing and the appeal, if there is one. Committed patients are also entitled to a regular review of the commitment, so they can't be held indefinitely.

In some states, civilly committed patients may be placed under the legal supervision of a hospital even after discharge. This is known as outpatient commitment. In this case, a patient can be returned to a hospital if he does not take prescribed medication or keep scheduled appointments. Again, outpatient commitments can happen only if the patient has a mental illness and is potentially dangerous as a result of that illness. Outpatient commitment is an area of some controversy in psychiatry. There is evidence that it may decrease use of emergency psychiatric services and may reduce the number of inpatient admissions for certain patients, but this finding is not consistent across jurisdictions. Also, there is concern that outpatient commitment may be used for patients who are competent to make treatment decisions and are not imminently dangerous.

Josh was very disorganized at the hearing, and he talked about the government and his need to protect the people. He didn't call any witnesses. The psychiatrist told the judge that Josh had attacked his roommate, was out of touch with reality, and remained symptomatic. He noted that Josh was finishing up a course of steroids for an awful episode of asthma, and that his bipolar disorder would likely be easier to control in a few days, when he was finished with the steroids. His parents were there, and they wanted him to sign in voluntarily. The hearing took about twenty minutes, and Josh was told he'd have to remain in the hospital for a little while longer.

A civil commitment only allows the hospital to keep the patient. It doesn't automatically mean that the patient is required to take medication. Involuntary medication is usually a separate procedural issue and involves hearing procedures similar to the commitment process. Again, to be treated with medication involuntarily, the patient must be both mentally ill and dangerous.

Josh didn't like being in the hospital. Other patients on the unit were disorganized and disruptive; he had no difficulty recognizing that *they* had mental problems. He didn't like the food. He didn't like that someone shined a flashlight on him every fifteen minutes during the night to record whether he was asleep or not. He knew this happened because he was awake much of the night. He didn't like going to group therapy or occupational therapy or medication education groups. Josh called his parents and complained. They were a bit confused about what to do. It was obvious that Josh needed help, but they also understood that he was unhappy and uncomfortable.

Josh's parents called the hospital administration and learned that there are agencies that inspect and accredit psychiatric hospitals to make sure conditions are appropriate for good treatment. When problems or conflicts occur between a patient and a hospital, many hospitals now have a patient liaison or patient rights adviser, a hospital employee whose job is to meet with patients to help them negotiate and resolve problems. For public psychiatric hospitals, the federal government is authorized to investigate alleged poor physical facilities or those with other issues related to patient health and safety. Passed in 1980, the Civil Rights for Institutionalized Persons Act (CRIPA) allows the government to pursue class action lawsuits to improve conditions in entire facilities or in public institutional systems such as psychiatric hospitals or correctional facilities.

In addition to this, most states have policy statements that document the rights of psychiatric patients. In some states, these rights are codified in state law. At the time of admission, psychiatric patients are given a document listing these rights, which are generally the following:

- the right to a clean and safe environment
- the right to be free from physical and emotional abuse
- the right to be informed about treatment options and to participate in the development of a treatment plan
- the right to make phone calls, receive mail, and have visitors
- the right to be free from unwarranted physical restraint or seclusion

There are often more rights than those listed here, but this is the basic minimum. Patients are allowed to have their own property, within reasonable limits. They may have, and wear, their own clothing. They may participate in religious services, if available. Psychiatric patients have a right to privacy, which means that if someone calls the unit looking for a patient, the unit clerk will not reveal the identity of patients on the unit. Clinical information is private as well and is shared only with people directly involved in the patient's care, such as the nursing staff or the unit social worker. Patients do have a right to their own clinical information, however. When Josh wanted to know what people were writing about him in his medical record, his doctor reviewed the record with him and explained the medical terminology in the notes. The doctor also explained Josh's diagnosis and the treatment options available to him. All of this information is available to psychiatric patients under most facilities' rights policies.

Rights can be restricted depending on the patient's clinical circumstances. For example, patients have a right to be free from physical restraint, but restraints may be used to preserve patient safety or the safety of others on the unit.

Patients have other responsibilities as well, and these are also included in the rights document. In general, psychiatric patients are responsible for telling their treatment team information that is relevant to their care and for behaving in compliance with the rules of the ward. Psychiatric inpatients must also interact with other patients in a safe and respectful fashion. Failure to do these things may make it difficult for a treatment team to provide the best care and may result in the patient's discharge from the hospital.

In later chapters, we talk more about what happens on an inpatient unit and about other areas where psychiatry intersects with the law.

Josh's mother tried to be supportive and helpful. When he complained about the food, she brought him meals he liked better, including his favorite take-out Chinese dish. When he complained about the other patients or the hospital routine, she listened. She told him about her own psychiatric hospitalization and how distressing that had been.

Josh was off his steroids soon. He took his mood stabilizer and a medication to treat the hallucinations and delusions. He was given another medication to help with sleep. Twelve days after Josh had charged at his roommate with a knife, he was much better and went home from the hospital. He didn't think he had anything to do with the government or television shows or plots to save or destroy America. He was sleeping normal hours and talking about things college students talk about. He left the hospital in time to go home for Thanksgiving and saw Dr. Smith for an appointment right after the holiday.

Josh didn't go back to school that semester. He'd been through a lot—the flu, a hospitalization for asthma, and a hospitalization for mania. He needed some time to recover, and the school wanted reassurance that he was not a danger to the community. He saw Dr. Smith regularly, his mood remained steady, and eventually he was able to return to college.

Chapter 3

The Brandt Family:
Why People Seek Care

THE BRANDT FAMILY was a large family with a lot going on. Sam and Alice adored all five of their adult children: Stuart, Richard, and the twins, Jack and Frank, were sons to be proud of. Their daughter, Becca, was charming one minute and difficult the next, but she was there when anyone needed her. As in any family, however, there were hard times, and people had their problems. We're borrowing the Brandt family to talk about some of the reasons people see psychiatrists.

We've already discussed how and where people get treatment for psychiatric disorders. The patients in our previous chapters all suffered from mood disorders. There are many other conditions that people seek care for—the current DSM-IV-TR lists 297 different disorders, and the fifth edition of the manual, due to be released in 2013, will list even more. In addition to mood disorders, the illnesses commonly seen by psychiatrists include schizophrenia, generalized anxiety disorder, panic attacks, obsessive-compulsive disorder, anorexia, and bulimia. These illnesses are included in the categories that psychiatrists think of as primary mental illnesses. The Brandt family members did not all have major mental illnesses, although they each suffered from serious difficulties. The DSM gives those problems names, or diagnoses, but we think of chronic and persistent mental illnesses a bit differently than we think about other problems. This distinction is, perhaps, artificial, and diagnosis may be influenced by forces outside the psychiatric community. Medical insurance will reimburse only for treatment of certain diagnoses, and disability insurance is available only to those with specific disorders. In addition, some programs and benefits are available only to people with diagnoses deemed to be "major mental illnesses."

Personality disorders can be terribly debilitating, but insurance will not usually pay for care if the patient's only diagnosis is a personality disorder. Substance abuse as a primary diagnosis is also segregated, and the treatment of drug and alcohol addictions, in the absence of other mental disorders, is *not* done in primary mental health facilities. Although the Brandts all had difficulties that have names, they did not all suffer from major mental illnesses.

Stuart was the oldest of the Brandt children, and he had always thought of himself as a strong person. He was the one his brothers and sister turned to when they had problems, and he quietly prided himself in his role as the shoulder that everyone cried on. He was the first one Sam and Alice called if they wanted an opinion on an investment or had a major decision to make. He was built like a linebacker, but he preferred playing his oboe to watching the Steelers. "Cerebral" was how Sam referred to his eldest son.

When Stuart's wife died unexpectedly in an accident at home, Stuart grieved and felt overwhelmed. His children did not do well either. It was horrible. Who wouldn't be distraught? For a while, he could barely eat, and nights were extremely hard; he was plagued with memories of Leslie, and he kept thinking that if he'd been home when she'd fallen, he would have gotten her to the hospital sooner, and she would have lived. The guilt was awful, and some nights he couldn't stop sobbing. He spoke to his priest, who offered comfort and reassurance, and his sister, Becca, came to stay with them for a while. Neighbors brought meals and invited the grieving family to dinner.

He appreciated everyone's support, but things only got worse. Stuart's younger brother Jack was diagnosed with lymphoma, and the family went through a period of feeling cursed. If that wasn't enough, Stuart's company went bankrupt, and he was laid off. Every time he thought his bad luck had run its course, something else happened.

Stuart became short tempered with his kids. He developed excruciating stomach pains. He lost a lot of weight, and he looked like a stranger to his friends and family. He saw his internist and a gastroenterologist, but neither could find any reason for his pain. They both attributed it to "stress" and offered sympathy after hearing all that had transpired. Becca insisted he needed help, and she scheduled an appointment for him with a psychiatrist.

"It's good to meet you," Dr. Smith said. "You sister told me on the phone that your family has been through a lot. She told me you lost your wife."

Stuart cried before he'd said a word. He helped himself to a tissue and tried to collect his thoughts.

"I didn't mean to upset you," Dr. Smith said.

"No, it's not you. It's just been awful," Stuart answered. He unfolded the events of the past six months, and the doctor listened.

"You have been through a great deal!" Dr. Smith sympathized. His response felt sincere to Stuart, not scripted. Stuart didn't know that as Dr. Smith listened, the psychiatrist's own personal losses flooded back at him. His mother had died of lymphoma when he was in medical school, and he still missed her. He remembered the awful time he'd had when he and his wife had separated briefly, and he couldn't imagine losing her forever. At one point, perhaps while Stuart talked about his little girl's despair, Dr. Smith consciously had to hold back his own tears. Could Stuart tell? He'd never know. Loss is a universal event, one we all relate to and empathize with. Dr. Smith was no exception.

The death of a close relative or friend, divorce or the end of a romantic relationship, workplace problems, or trouble coping with illness or financial problems are common stresses that can lead to psychiatric symptoms. People sometimes have difficulties if they've had to relocate, or after any major upheavals, such as those caused by fire or natural disasters. Other common reasons people seek professional help include distress after being the victim of a crime, or when there are difficult family dynamics. Stress, in and of itself, may cause both physical and psychological symptoms, or it can cause a psychiatric illness. Some people deal with stress well; others do not.

In Stuart's situation, the stress level might drive anyone to an extreme state, and his short temper, stomach pains, and even his weight loss seem understandable to an outsider hearing his horrible story. His symptoms may be *understandable*, but nevertheless, they were distressing and disabling to Stuart.

Grief looks a lot like major depression: people become sad and tearful, have trouble sleeping, and lose their appetites. It can be a struggle to get through the days, and it can be hard to feel any pleasure. Psychiatrists may have a difficult time telling when normal grief has turned to major depression, though if someone is suicidal or psychotic, or if grief continues to interfere with a person's ability to function for a long time, a psychiatrist may diagnose an illness and prescribe medications in addition to psychotherapy.

It's never normal to hallucinate or to suffer from delusions. People who are bereaved may experience vivid verbal memories of their loved one, such as hearing the person call their name or seeing them sitting in their favorite chair. These are not pathological hallucinations but a normal part of bereavement. The experience of grief is shaped by culture, and this always needs to be considered during the psychiatric evaluation. Bereaved patients may also have fleeting thoughts of giving up or not being able to go on following a death, but persistent thoughts of suicide are never normal, and these people need to seek help.

One of the dividing lines used to determine if a person's reaction to stress, particularly due to loss, is within the range of normal reactions is the issue of seeking care. People don't typically come to a psychiatrist when they are grieving. Instead, they seek the comfort of family, friends, and their religious leaders. Everyone expects to feel bad after a death, and people don't typically think they need professional help, nor should they. Once someone defines himself as a patient, or when other people in his life insist there is a problem, the situation is a little different. Either the symptoms are extreme or the person's behavior is problematic in some way. In Stuart's case, every time he turned around, another blow was dealt, and he'd developed excruciating stomach pains and distressing personality changes.

Stress can cause any psychiatric disorder in someone who is susceptible to a specific psychiatric illness. People with a predisposition can become depressed or manic; those with schizophrenia may have an acute episode; and people with anxiety disorders may get worse. It seems counterintuitive that someone dealing with a loss can become manic, but this happens.

Stress can make other medical conditions worse as well—ulcers, migraine headaches, asthma, irritable bowel syndrome, and pre-existing pain syndromes are all illnesses that can get worse. The hormones released by stress can have negative effects on the body, particularly the immune system, and can make people more susceptible to illnesses and infections. Stuart's abdominal pains were totally new, and a medical workup was absolutely necessary.

Stress, loss, and painful events are part of life. Although stress may cause suffering and make physical and psychiatric symptoms worse, it's important to note that just because someone has had an episode of a psychiatric disorder, all stresses will not necessarily lead to a relapse. There are people who have been ill and who have recovered, who are extremely resilient and hold up well under the worst of circumstances. Stress can lead to disorder, but it doesn't always, even in people who are predisposed. Unless personal history dictates otherwise, people who have had a past episode of mental illness are not necessarily constitutionally fragile.

The first thing Stuart needed was for someone to listen to his problems with a caring ear. His wife's death was sudden, unexpected, and tragic. He'd held his family together and coped with the loss of his job, his brother's cancer, and his children's grief. Dr. Smith commented on how hard this must have been.

"You'd think I'd be able to suck it up," Stuart said.

"Is that what people are telling you?" Dr. Smith asked.

"No. Actually, everyone's been pretty sympathetic. Everyone else is having a rough time, too. Jack is having all these treatments, and I feel like I'm one more drain on everyone's reserves. But, no. No one says I should suck it up."

Stuart needed the ongoing support of his family, friends, and religious community, and he got that. Did he need medication? Maybe. It might help with his sadness, irritability, and appetite and weight loss. His stomach pains were severe, and all his tests were negative. Sometimes pain syndromes get better with psychiatric medications. The psychiatrist who saw Stuart also urged him to come for psychotherapy.

Stuart's story certainly made sense. Let's a try a scenario that's not as clear.

Stuart's brother Jack had a more complicated story. Jack felt victimized by his boss, and he was preoccupied with his problems at work; it was really all he talked about, and everyone in his life was tired of listening. He called his mother, Alice, every day, and finally she told him to get some help.

Jack went to a psychiatrist with a chief complaint that he had trouble dealing with stress at work. He had no history of mental illness. His perception was that the boss was the problem, and so his problem was caused by something external to him: stress. Life got hard.

Jack was a very successful businessman and had been with his current company for eight years. He believed that his boss was part of a group conspiring to harm him. The boss, according to Jack, had bugged his phone and offered him a poisoned doughnut. Sometimes he heard voices, and the details of his concerns didn't really make sense. He talked about objects being moved on his desk, and he couldn't say why his boss might do this or what exactly it meant. He acted very strangely, and everyone was worried about him. Sometimes he prayed loudly at work, something he'd never done before. Jack had lost seven pounds, and sometimes his right arm started to shake for no reason. This had all been going on for the past two months, and his mother hadn't just suggested he see a psychiatrist—she had scheduled the appointment, and both she and Sam went with him.

Jack thought his problem was the behavior of his boss, but he did not have an understandable reaction to a stressful situation. There was no reason to believe that the boss was poisoning him, and this didn't explain the voices Jack heard. He needed a medical workup to discover why he was suddenly psychotic. The episodes during which his arm shook sounded like focal seizures. The psychiatrist was very worried and sent him to see a neurologist. A brain scan revealed a tumor, and this is how Jack's lymphoma was diagnosed.

Difficult life circumstances can cause a variety of problems. The first thing a psychiatrist must do is take a complete history and figure out if the patient's perception of external stress is the cause of the problem, or if other factors might be involved. There is a lot for a psychiatrist to think about in the interaction between stress and the reactions people have to it.

Becca Brandt was an engaging young woman who loved to be with people. Conversation came naturally to her, and Becca made friends easily. Her laugh was infectious, her smile beguiling. People were drawn to Becca, even captivated by her, but then something happened. A friend might do something that rubbed Becca the wrong way—maybe she was too busy to go out when Becca really wanted to, or maybe she expressed an opinion Becca found objectionable. Suddenly the friend was no longer a friend. Associates were idealized one moment and vilified the next. People, Becca would announce with an air of indignation, always let her down. Even her family relied on her much too much, and her brothers only called when they needed her help.

She liked to be out and about, and when she was alone, Becca felt miserable and desperate. Sometimes, she drank to ease the loneliness. Other times, she took a razor and sliced the skin on the inside of her arms. She didn't want to die, but something about the sting of the blade and the sight of her blood was reassuring. Becca was vivacious and lively when she was with new people, but the people who knew her well often felt Becca was just too much work.

What about disorders of the personality? What does that even mean, and is it a useful way of looking at people and their problems?

People have personalities: characteristic ways of behaving and responding. They have styles; they have flair. Some people are introverted and prefer the familiar; others are extroverted and like a changing flow of stimulation. Some are easy to get along with; others have trouble holding on to friends. People can be very impulsive, or they can ruminate over every small decision. These characteristics, however, occur on a continuum, and few people fall entirely within the description of a single personality type. We talk about personality in terms of traits. When someone's personality causes significant problems, we talk about personality in terms of disorder.

There are eight personality disorders in the current DSM-IV-TR. This will certainly change in the DSM-V because a major reconsideration of personality assessment is in progress. For now, personality disorders are listed in clusters: cluster A includes three disorders deemed odd or eccentric. Cluster B disorders are the more dramatic, impulsive, and erratic personality types: narcissistic, borderline, antisocial, and histrionic. Cluster C consists of the more anxious and fearful personality types. Becca is an example of someone with a cluster B personality disorder.

Someone's personality is considered to be disordered when her style of behaving interferes with her ability to function or causes her significant subjective distress. The designation is a matter of opinion, and there's no absolute line that divides normal from disordered. It has to be a problem over a long period, in a variety of settings—someone who has trouble getting along with a particular neighbor, or working for a certain company, does not have a personality disorder if his style works for him in other settings.

Many people who meet criteria for a personality disorder do not come to treatment to have their personalities fixed per se. For example, people with schizoid personality disorder are not interested in social relationships and tend toward solitary activities. They don't like being with people, and they don't generally see this as a problem or seek help to change it. By definition, they prefer being alone and are not troubled by their lack of relationships. People with this personality type come for treatment only if they have another psychiatric disorder, such as a mood or an anxiety problem.

Often, people with more dramatic personalities, like Becca, come for help because they become overwhelmed by the situations they get into. They often do not see their own role in creating their difficulties.

Personality disorders are frequently diagnosed in difficult and demanding patients, often those in the cluster B (dramatic and impulsive) realm who, like Becca, may stir up the emotions of people around them, including their psychiatrists! Sometimes the reference to a personality disorder means, more specifically, borderline personality disorder. People with borderline personality disorder have symptoms that include instability in their moods, difficulty controlling their impulses, problems with their sense of identity, and a tendency to see people in their lives as all good or all bad. On psychiatric units, patients with this style often engage the staff in ways that lead the treatment team to take sides, a process called *splitting*. These patients may also engage in alarming self-destructive behaviors, and they are frequently suicidal. Patients with borderline personality disorder often have a co-occurring mood disorder, and they may also have difficulties with substance abuse, anxiety, eating disorders, or other problems of impulse control, such as shoplifting or gambling.

Certainly, there are people who behave in ways that put others off: they are too rigid, too dramatic, or too bizarre to sustain ongoing relationships. Sometimes it's helpful to be able to explain someone's difficulties with a label, simply because people are comforted by the explanatory nature of a diagnosis. In the case of personality disorders, the diagnosis is more descriptive. It does not tell us the etiology—or cause—of the problem, and often it does not guide treatment. Some personality disorders have no clearly effective treatments.

There is a pejorative edge to saying someone has a personality disorder—it's sometimes a way of saying they are difficult to treat or even unlikeable. Sometimes the diagnosis is inadvertently given when there is a personality conflict between the clinician and the patient. If such a conflict is an isolated event, and not representative of other relationships the patient has, then the diagnosis is a mistake.

When a patient has a mental illness, such as schizophrenia or depression or bipolar disorder, she is perceived as the victim of an awful disease. When someone has a personality disorder, she is seen as being the cause of her own problems. People can be demanding, especially those suffering physical or mental anguish, and the personality disorder label sometimes creates a prejudice against them. Although personality disorders are categorized as mental illnesses, they are coded separately, and insurance does not reimburse for their treatment unless another disorder is present.

Psychiatry does not have a cohesive way of approaching these disorders, and among ourselves, their validity is unclear. The diagnostic criteria for antisocial personality disorder includes repeated disregard for the law and repeated physical fights or aggression. How, one might wonder, does someone with this psychiatric illness differ from a common criminal? And why do we call this a mental illness? When is someone deemed schizoid or avoidant versus just plain shy?

The treatment for personality disorders is psychotherapy, and it is not always clear how helpful this is, or when it may be harmful. Certainly, pushing fragile people to discuss painful past events can be detrimental. Studies show that certain types of therapy can be helpful to people with borderline personality disorder, but there is not much evidence that psychotherapy cures personality disorders. "Cure" is a funny word when talking about personalities. Psychotherapy may help people gain insight into their patterns of reacting, and it may help dissipate anger and anguish that fuel troublesome reactions. Sometimes, psychotherapy offers a measure of comfort and relief. It's more about helping someone with personality problems learn to negotiate the world within the context of who she is than it is about changing the essence of her being.

One of the concerns with a personality disorder diagnosis is that it may close the door on diagnostic thinking, and other diagnoses may be missed. Mood instability is a prominent symptom of borderline personality disorder, and the treatment is different if one views the problem as a primary disorder of mood rather than a primary disorder of personality. Some mood disorder specialists assert that the chaotic emotions and behaviors of borderline patients are better explained as symptoms of a bipolar disorder variant; when these patients are given mood stabilizers, they feel better, and their behavior becomes less disruptive.

Traumatic past events, especially during the formative years of childhood, may play a role in the development of these difficulties, and posttraumatic stress disorder can be a useful way of thinking about these problems. It's certainly a less stigmatizing and more sympathetic way to view someone who has been through horrible things. The role of early trauma in the development of personality disorders remains unclear. Many people with these disorders were abused as children, but this is not a clear cause-and-effect relationship. Not everyone with a personality disorder was abused, and not everyone who was abused develops a personality disorder. Some therapists have believed that if a patient had a borderline personality, they *must* have been abused. Patients were encouraged to "uncover" memories of the abuse, which must have occurred and must have been repressed. It is now considered bad practice to encourage patients to believe things happened that they do not readily remember on their own.

People come for help when their personalities get in the way of their lives, sometimes coming in of their own accord, sometimes at the request or mandate of others. Often, they don't see themselves as the problem; rather, they feel victimized by the outside world. There is a lot we don't know about both the causes and treatments of personality disorders, and this remains a weakness in our field.

Alice urged Becca to go see a psychiatrist.

"I don't need a psychiatrist!" Becca said.

"That's what Stuart said," Alice reminded Becca, "and you were the one who found that nice doctor who helped him."

Becca went once. She didn't like Dr. Smith. He asked too many questions, and he didn't really listen, or so Becca said. Alice was exasperated with her daughter. She'd met Dr. Smith and thought he was nice and very concerned. He was the one who had realized that Jack needed a brain scan! Stuart had found him to be extremely helpful. How could Becca not like him? What was there not to like? What Becca didn't tell her mother was that Dr. Smith had suggested she stop drinking—that when she drank, she was more susceptible to feeling down and to injuring herself. He also suggested that a medication might be helpful, and Becca didn't want to hear that she needed "strong drugs." She didn't want to stop drinking, and she didn't want to take medicines. For now, she wasn't going back to Dr. Smith or to any other psychiatrist.

Every night, after his wife, Linda, went to bed, Richard Brandt, the youngest of the Brandt brothers, would turn on the computer and surf. He told himself he was just going to catch up on the headlines, and he would start on Drudge Report and CNN, but as the night progressed, he always drifted over to pornography sites. His tastes were very specific, and he knew where to find exactly what he wanted. He watched videos, he looked at photos, and he went to a site where people posted their sexual fantasies. Linda would never understand. Even Richard didn't really understand why he did this when he could just have sex with his wife. At some point, late into the night, Richard would masturbate. Then he'd clear the computer's history and go to bed. Linda would wake up when he got into bed, and some nights she wanted sex, but Richard was not interested. He was sexually satisfied. He always felt guilty and promised himself that he would never do it again. And yet, the next night he would be back in front of the computer.

People struggle with all types of behaviors, some we might even call addictive or compulsive, or resulting from poor impulse control. Richard should have just stopped looking at pornography. His behavior left him drenched in guilt, and it harmed his marriage.

We can change the scenario a little. We can rewrite it so that Richard drank until he was intoxicated, or shot heroin through his veins. We could take him out of the house and have him expose himself to strangers, or we could watch him gamble until he was tens of thousands of dollars in debt. Richard could eat a third pint of mocha chip ice cream when he was morbidly obese and suffering from heart disease and diabetes, or he could simply light up yet one more cigarette, even though it aggravated his emphysema. While it's not illegal to smoke cigarettes or eat too much ice cream, and it is illegal to shoot heroin and to expose oneself, these behaviors all have something in common. The person who engages in them often feels an uncomfortable compulsion to do so; he can't, or won't, simply stop because that's the right thing to do, or because it's illegal or ultimately harmful to himself or others. Richard enjoyed an activity that might have disastrous consequences, but he was unable to stop.

Psychiatry struggles with how to even categorize these disorders of behavior. In everyday parlance, they are probably best described as addictions, though many people reserve that term for chemical dependencies (meaning drugs and alcohol) that cause a physical addiction. There is no such physical addiction to gambling, sexual behaviors, overeating, or many of the other behaviors we think of loosely as addictions. In 2007, the American Psychiatric Association looked at whether to include "video game addiction" as a diagnosable disorder and decided it should not be considered a mental illness.

One of the reasons we struggle with how to classify these disorders is that it's not completely clear to us how much these problems are caused by mental illnesses and how much they are linked to poor self-discipline. Certainly there is a continuum. If we look at alcoholism, one of the more common addictions, we can see clear evidence of a genetic predisposition.

We used the term compulsive because Richard felt compelled to look at pornography, and he became anxious and uncomfortable when he tried to resist. These behaviors, however, are not considered by psychiatrists to be in the same category as those we term obsessive-compulsive disorder. These difficulties are considered disorders of behavior. The symptoms we associate with obsessive-compulsive disorder—repeated checking, washing, counting, hoarding, and ritualistic behavior—are a type of anxiety disorder. Richard's problem is behavioral. If this sounds confusing, that's because it is!

Richard went to see Dr. Smith for help because he struggled with his guilt and his distress at being out of control. He worried that his behavior would ruin his marriage if his wife discovered what he was doing. People with behavioral difficulties, however, often do not identify them as problems. More often, they come for help because they've run into obstacles, often with the law, perhaps with their families or their employers, and their distress is more about the consequences of the behavior than about a desire to stop. Few alcoholics want to quit drinking until they have problems with their health, the law, their employers, or their loved ones.

We don't understand what causes and maintains these disorders, and our treatments offer limited success: they help some of the people some of the time. Insight-oriented psychotherapy does not usually cure these behaviors when it is the only treatment given. Self-help groups, such as Narcotics Anonymous, are extremely helpful to many people. They provide guidance, a plan, and support, and they hold individuals accountable for their behaviors in ways that can be invaluable. In recent years, there have been more medications to treat these conditions. Examples include methadone, buprenorphine, and naltrexone for narcotic addictions, nicotine patches for smokers, and hormonal agents for those with overpowering and deviant sexual drives.

What does a psychiatrist like Dr. Smith think about when a patient like Richard comes for treatment? First, he considers whether other diagnoses are contributing to the patient's difficulties, and here there were none. People can become hypersexual during an episode of mania, but Richard was not manic. Dr. Smith considered whether medications might help, but no medications "treat" a married man's desire to look at pornography. Dr. Smith thought about whether psychotherapy might be helpful to Richard, and this was a complicated issue. It used to be thought that if a patient could understand the underlying meaning of a behavior, he could control it. We now know that this is not generally the case, and insight-oriented psychotherapy does not stop compulsive behaviors. It may, however, help a patient deal with his guilt, identify triggers that leave him vulnerable, or provide an arena for accountability, and these may be helpful. We don't, however, tell someone who smokes or eats too much that they need in-depth psychotherapy; instead we recommend programs (like Weight Watchers) that target specific behaviors. At the same time, Dr. Smith did not tell Richard, "I'm sorry, there's nothing I can do for you, and you'll always be addicted to pornography," because that's not true. What he also did not say was, "I promise that if you come for regular psychotherapy sessions that you'll never look at pornography and you'll have a great sex life with your wife." There was a lot to *not* say!

Some people conquer troublesome behaviors on their own, and we don't know why one person can give up smoking cold turkey while another wakes every morning with an unsuccessful vow to stop. We assume that a person's genetic makeup dictates at least some of his vulnerabilities to alcohol or drugs. We don't know what steers a person's sexual desires. Perhaps it is the intrinsic push-pull of the addiction that makes treatment so tenuous: Richard wants to stop, but ultimately, he finds his addiction pleasurable.

Richard saw Dr. Smith for regular psychotherapy sessions, and at one point, he tried taking a medication for anxiety. The medicine had the side effect of decreasing his sex drive, but not enough to interfere with his sexual compulsion. Richard was not willing to try a self-help group for people with sexual addictions, and eventually he stopped going to treatment. If asked if therapy had been helpful, Richard would say it had been; however, the treatment did not decrease his interest in pornography.

Frank Brandt, Jack's twin, finished the marathon and was happy that he broke his personal record. Training had taken the better part of six months and occupied every spare moment of his off-duty time. Although his work didn't suffer, Frank's girlfriend made offhand comments about his inability to commit to anything but his running shoes. His fellow police officers admired his stamina but questioned his sanity and teased him by putting cupcakes in his locker. One day, not long after the marathon, during his usual five-mile run, Frank was overwhelmed by crushing chest pain. He managed to get home, but by the time his girlfriend met him at the door, the pain was gone. He laughed it off as "old man's hypochondria" since it had happened on the eve of his fortieth birthday. He told his partner, Tavon, what happened and mentioned in passing that if he ever had to live like one of those "cardiac cripples," he'd rather just shoot himself. Tavon had just completed his suicide prevention training and promptly told his supervisor that Frank had made a reference to suicide. Frank was shocked when his lieutenant called him in and referred him to the employee assistance program.

Frank had made an offhand comment that led to a mental health evaluation. He never seriously meant to kill himself. He wasn't depressed, and he didn't expect his statement to cause concern on the job. Fortunately, nothing bad happened to Frank. He saw the police psychologist, a former army captain with a pleasantly twisted sense of humor, and unexpectedly ended up telling him all about his girlfriend and the issues in their relationship.

"But I wouldn't kill myself," Frank said. "My family's had enough going on. I was the donor for my brother Jack's stem cell transplant, and my sister-in-law fell off a stepladder, hit her head, and died. The last thing I want is to be one more dead person in my family!"

The psychologist convinced Frank to see his family physician for a cardiac examination, and he listened attentively to Frank's problems.

Statements about suicide may be made sarcastically or out of exasperation, and the intent is not always clear. It may be up to friends or colleagues like Tavon to decide if and when to intervene. Tavon was cautious because he knew Frank carried a gun and was having relationship difficulties. A statement about suicide in that context was particularly concerning. In this case, there was a simple miscommunication.

Sometimes people seek care, or are referred for care, because of suicidal statements or actual suicide attempts. Suicidal thoughts or a suicide attempt may be the final straw that compels someone to seek treatment. People without mental illnesses may impulsively injure themselves during a temporary state of distress after something bad happens. An example of this might be a teenager who overdoses after a romantic breakup but who really does not want to die.

Sometimes a person is suicidal as a symptom of mental illness. People don't usually think of psychiatric illnesses as being fatal diseases, but they can be. Major depression, bipolar disorder, schizophrenia, and anorexia all have significant mortality rates. Even with treatment, the risk of dying from suicide still exists, although at a lower level than if it is left untreated. According to the Centers for Disease Control, there are about ninety suicides every day in the United States, or one every sixteen minutes.

Suicide takes a heavy toll on many people, including the family members, friends, and co-workers of the deceased. At the same time, people have trouble understanding why it happened and how to offer comfort. When someone dies from a terminal illness, there may be a sense of relief that their suffering has ended. A death from murder allows survivors to displace their grief into anger at the perpetrator. Sudden accidental deaths or deaths from natural disaster are often accompanied by an outpouring of support from the community. Suicide is different. Friends may have trouble knowing what to say or may even wonder if they should mention the death at all.

The suicide act itself may be an expression of hostility, especially if committed in the survivors' presence or in a way designed for others to discover the body. A suicide note may explain the trigger for the event or document just how psychiatrically ill the person was prior to his death, but in two-thirds of suicide deaths, no note is left. Survivors are left to speculate and to anguish over what signs they missed or what more they could have done. This is particularly true if the victim was not known to have a history of mental illness, or if the death was a high-profile media event like a murder-suicide.

Professionals who study suicide and its prevention are called suicidologists. Suicidologists have tried to figure out the many causes by defining categories. The term *anomic suicide* refers to a suicide committed by someone who thinks the world has become such a lawless and chaotic place that it's not worth living in. The term *rational suicide* is used to refer to a suicide committed by someone who is not mentally ill but who prefers death to living an intolerable life. An example of this would be a death row inmate who volunteers for execution rather than serve a life term in a maximum security prison. Another example would be someone who jumps from a burning building. Finally, terminally ill people may believe that suicide is a means of choosing the time and manner of their own death. Two states have passed laws allowing physician-assisted suicide for terminally ill, mentally competent patients.

Society's view of this act has changed quite a bit over the years. In the Middle Ages, suicide was a crime punished by the confiscation of the deceased's property, and the deceased was banned from burial in holy ground because suicide was considered an unforgivable sin. Today, we know that in most cases, suicide is the result of mental illness. Other risk factors include an active substance abuse problem, the presence of a personality disorder, previous attempts, and a recent stressor, such as the loss of a job or a relationship. Young people between the ages of 10 and 24 are at increased risk, as are people over the age of 65 who suffer from chronic medical conditions. Married people and people with religious affiliations are less likely to commit suicide.

Suicide prevention programs were developed to increase public awareness of the problem. Programs have been developed for middle schools and high schools, colleges, correctional facilities, and the military. They generally involve distributing information about suicide and how to access mental health services. Prevention programs teach people to recognize signs of clinical depression and how to talk about suicide with those at risk. In 1999, the surgeon general recognized suicide as a significant national public health problem and called for nationwide intervention. By 2001, twenty-five states had statewide prevention plans, and many had school-based services for at-risk adolescents.

There is also help available for the survivors. We've already talked about the value of therapy for the treatment of bereavement and the use of medication for complicated bereavement. The American Foundation for Suicide Prevention carries an up-to-date list of online and local support groups at www.afsp.org.

Meeting with the police force psychologist changed Frank's life. He'd been thinking about retiring, and he decided to go back to school and become a mental health professional. He'd never had mental health issues of his own, but he watched from the sidelines as Stuart, Richard, and his twin brother, Jack, all felt they got something out of seeing Dr. Smith. And he felt the frustration of watching Becca continue in her troubled ways. Frank had gotten some interesting insights from seeing the police force psychologist, and he decided to go into personal psychotherapy as he changed vocations.

There are those who say that everyone can benefit from psychotherapy. This is an extrapolation of Socrates's proclamation, "The unexamined life is not worth living." There are others who joke that Prozac should be added, like fluoride, to the water supply. These are ways of pointing out both how helpful treatment can be and how ubiquitous distress is.

We've talked about people who come to treatment for issues related to illness, symptoms, distress, and dysfunction. There are also people who see psychiatrists for psychotherapy as a way of gaining a better understanding of themselves in the absence of a psychiatric disorder. They may be looking to gain insight into their personalities and motivations as a goal of its own, and often they look to psychoanalysts, or those who practice psychodynamically oriented psychotherapy, for treatment.

Perhaps the people most likely to enter psychotherapy as part of an introspective process are those who are training to be psychotherapists themselves. Psychoanalysts are required to undergo a personal analysis as part of their training. The analyst must have an understanding of his own unconscious conflicts in order to help his patients.

At one point, psychotherapy, and especially psychoanalysis, was considered necessary for would-be psychiatrists, but now there is no consensus statement about whether personal therapy is a necessary step to becoming a psychiatrist. Many supervisors continue to encourage their trainees to undergo psychotherapy, especially if the psychiatrist plans to use psychotherapy as a treatment for his own patients. This may be helpful for several reasons.

A surgeon-in-training can watch a surgery. He can perform one with a more experienced surgeon in the room, and any given surgical procedure is finished within hours. Psychotherapy, however, is often regarded as private, and it is a process over time, sometimes years, so teaching it can be difficult. Supervision generally relies on the student's accounts of what was said because supervisors do not typically observe the sessions. Being a psychotherapy patient is one of the few ways in which a therapist gets to see what goes on behind closed doors. And while we certainly don't believe that it's necessary for every doctor to experience every illness or treatment to render good care, many believe that spending some time in the role of the patient helps a doctor to empathize. It is also useful for the therapist to be aware of his own motivations and concerns. We talk more about this in the next chapter.

Since we brought up the issue of people seeking treatment for education and insight, we'll end by addressing the question of whether all psychiatrists are crazy. Forgive us for using such a derogatory term, but that's the stereotype that travels. Simply put, psychiatrists are people, and they deviate, like all people, from any image of "normal." Some psychiatrists have psychiatric disorders, others have family members with psychiatric disorders, and some have no personal connection to mental illness. In any field, there are people who have a personal interest in the diseases they treat, often because of family history or personal experience. One might also ask if psychiatrists are more likely to have idiosyncratic personality styles, but there is no research into this.

We believe there is no shame in seeking psychiatric care, and we wish everyone believed it. Perhaps part of the human condition is that we are all vulnerable, that human beings have problems, and that life certainly has its rough patches. People get sick, physically and mentally, and they get better. It's unfortunate that the stigma of mental illness keeps people from seeking care for things that so often get better with a little intervention and attention.

Chapter 4

Tara:
Let's Talk

AT ONE O'CLOCK every Thursday, Tara Jackson went to see Dr. Philip Linus. She usually arrived a few minutes early and while she waited, Tara leafed through a magazine or listened to music on her iPod. On the hour, Dr. Linus would open the door, and Tara would follow him into his office. He was a tall man with salt-and-pepper hair, and he always greeted her with the exact same expression. It's hard to characterize just what his expression said—it wasn't quite enthusiastic, but it wasn't bland either.

In his office, it would be just the two of them alone together. Perhaps Dr. Linus would ask how Tara was doing, or perhaps he would simply wait for her to begin speaking.

On one visit, Tara told Dr. Linus all the important things that had happened in her life over the course of the week. She had finished a project at work and was relieved when it was done. She had stayed up late several nights to meet the deadline. Her father had been annoyed that Tara had talked on her Blackberry at midnight.

Up until now, Dr. Linus had simply listened. When Tara mentioned her father, his eyes got a little bigger. She talked about her father often. Their relationship was difficult.

"This bothered you," Dr. Linus said. It was partly a statement and partly a question.

"He treats me like a child who should have a nine o'clock bedtime."

She was a petite woman, just over five feet tall, who looked significantly younger than her 26 years. Dark bangs covered Tara's forehead, and she had piercing blue eyes. She was burdened with responsibility at both home and work, so while she looked like a teenager, she seemed somehow old for her age. She always wore a suit and pumps, and she was rapidly climbing the corporate ladder. Not surprisingly, Tara had already been treated for an ulcer.

Dr. Linus commented on the bind she and her father were in: they might all be more comfortable if she moved out, but Tara's parents needed her there. Tara felt controlled by her father. She lived in his house, and he expected her to follow his rules, but she felt like a prisoner. She could afford to get her own place, and she mentioned this whenever her father complained, but without her financial contribution, her parents couldn't afford to pay their own bills. At least that is what they told her. Tara's mother didn't drive, and her parents often asked for her help with errands and appointments.

Dr. Linus wondered if it had always been this way, and Tara said yes. Her father wanted her close—he demanded it, actually—but when she didn't do things his way, he got angry and insisted she was a burden. He had done this all through her high school years—he wouldn't let her go out with her friends and then got mad when she watched TV or talked on the phone.

Dr. Linus listened. He pointed out patterns in her thinking and behavior when he noticed them, and he challenged her insistent belief that she couldn't possibly move out of the house. As he listened, he thought about patients he'd seen in the past with similar stories. He thought, too, about his own daughter and wondered if she'd ever grow into a pretty young woman who resented him.

Soon Dr. Linus let Tara know that it was time for the session to end, and she asked for a refill on her medication. He wrote the prescription and saw her to the door.

"See you next week," Tara said.

There is much to say about psychotherapy, and many books have been written about different kinds of therapies. A search for "psychotherapy" on the Amazon.com website reveals more than 75,000 results! But what is it? What gets said behind the closed door, and why does it work?

Psychotherapy is a treatment in which the talking itself is what helps the patient get better. Each type of psychotherapy is associated with a

theory of how patients develop their problems, and the content of the
therapy—what the doctor and the patient talk about—is different depending on the type of therapy being done. Most therapies have certain
parameters, such as the length and frequency of the session, treatment
goals, and an agenda for what the patient and therapist talk about in a
session. Each therapy also has a duration, which may be many weeks, if
not months or years. All therapy is grounded in confidentiality, unless
the psychiatrist is worried that the patient is imminently dangerous. This
certainly wasn't the case during Tara's session with Dr. Linus. Finally,
there is a tacit agreement that the patient will not keep secrets from the
therapist.

When Tara first went to see Dr. Linus, she hadn't been sure what to
expect. She had a friend who saw a psychiatrist, but he had only fifteen-
minute visits every six weeks or so, and she didn't think he could be talking about much in that short time. And in fact, every meeting with a
psychiatrist is not a therapy session. Tara's friend was being seen only for
medication management. Tara's psychiatrist wanted her to come weekly
for fifty-minute psychotherapy sessions.

The distinction between a medication management appointment and
a psychotherapy session is sometimes blurred. Suppose during a medication management appointment, the doctor asks, "How are you?" and the
patient starts talking about a stressful circumstance in his life. Perhaps the
psychiatrist offers some suggestions, or perhaps the patient feels helped
simply by talking briefly about his situation. This encounter was therapeutic for the patient even though the brief session wasn't intended to be
for therapy.

Similarly, even with irregular or infrequent sessions, some patients are
able to use treatment to make substantial changes. Many people want sessions every other week or once a month because they can't afford more
frequent sessions, or they can't logistically make the time in their lives.
Other people don't want regularly scheduled sessions at all, and they call
when they'd like to come for an appointment. The frequency of sessions
may vary with how the patient is feeling and how things are going in his
life. They may also vary with the doctor's therapeutic orientation, or with
how flexible the psychiatrist is able to be with her schedule.

For the sake of a definition, psychiatrists usually agree that sessions need to occur with some regularity and last for at least twenty-five minutes to be called psychotherapy. Traditionally, psychotherapy sessions last for fifty minutes, and the patient comes once or twice a week. Shorter sessions are for pharmacologic management and usually focus more on illness assessment and medication issues, and less on looking at either the patterns in the patient's life or the issues that come up in the relationship between the doctor and the patient.

When Tara had first come to see Dr. Linus, she hadn't known if she needed psychotherapy. Psychotherapies can be classified as *insight-oriented* psychotherapy, including psychoanalysis, and *supportive* psychotherapy. *Cognitive-behavioral therapy* (CBT) is a specific type of therapy that is based on the idea that feelings and behaviors are learned or conditioned responses to environmental stimuli.

Psychoanalysis is the oldest form of formal psychotherapy and dates back to the late nineteenth century. In the 1950s and 1960s, many therapists branded their own forms of treatment, for example, rational emotive therapy, gestalt therapy, transactional analysis, and therapies based on existential philosophies. Many of these treatments are no longer widely used or available, so we will focus instead on the more common divisions of treatment.

Insight-oriented therapy is about introspection and revolves around the theory that a person's actions and feelings are influenced by their past experiences. It assumes the existence of an unconscious mind, meaning that people are influenced by forces in their psyche that they are not aware of, and that by exploring their past, their fantasies, and even their dreams, they can learn about their unconscious.

The most intensive insight-oriented psychotherapy is psychoanalysis. In psychoanalysis, the patient comes for therapy four or five times a week, and treatment lasts for an average of six years. During a psychoanalysis, the patient lies on a couch and does not look at the psychoanalyst. This treatment is expensive and time-consuming, and while many people find it beneficial, the use of psychoanalysis as a treatment for mental illness is not scientifically proven beneficial, perhaps because it's so difficult to do prospective outcome studies; we talk more below about why this is. Its use is limited by the cost, the time investment, and the availability of other, faster-acting and proven treatments. It is used today as a means of gaining personal insight, for educational purposes, and sometimes to address personality pathology, often in conjunction with medications. Tara's psychotherapy was not psychoanalysis: she went only once a week; she didn't lie on a couch; and Dr. Linus was not specifically trained as a psychoanalyst. Although it was not psychoanalysis, it was a psychodynamic treatment derived from some of the principals used in psychoanalysis.

In supportive therapy, the emphasis is not on exploring the past, but on helping the patient to deal with present circumstances. Traditionally, it was seen as an inferior form of psychotherapy, reserved for sicker patients who were deemed more fragile than the more articulate, educated, and curious patients who were felt to be the best candidates for an explorative, insight-oriented therapy. A good psychotherapist is able to use both supportive and insight-oriented techniques with some flexibility depending on the needs of the patient at the moment.

Cognitive-behavioral psychotherapy is a type of supportive treatment through which patients explore their patterns of thinking and behaving. The emphasis is on current symptoms, and the focus of treatment is to look at what events and thoughts precede uncomfortable feelings and behaviors. CBT is used to treat anxiety disorders and depression. The therapist may take a more active role in guiding the agenda, and patients are often asked to do homework. The treatment may be limited to a specific number of sessions and is conducted over weeks or months, not years. Sometimes, in the treatment of phobias, the therapist may see the patient in settings other than an office. A patient who is too anxious to drive across bridges, for example, might be accompanied by her therapist while she drives over a bridge.

Why was Tara told she needed therapy while her friend was seen only for brief visits to address his symptoms and medications? Was Tara sicker? Is this why she needed more care?

If someone goes to the doctor with symptoms of a urinary tract infection, a culture is done, a species of bacteria is isolated, and an antibiotic is prescribed for a set amount of time—it's the same for every patient and every doctor. Psychiatry is not like this. We have practice guidelines that define diagnostic entities and medication regimens for treatment. What we don't have are clear guidelines on which problems need psychotherapy, which type of psychotherapy, and for how long. We know a little, and so it's possible that Tara and her friend had completely different issues and therefore got completely different treatments. Psychiatrists, however, place varying emphasis on their use of psychotherapy, and treatment is often determined by the doctor's orientation. Tara could have seen another doctor who would have prescribed medications for panic attacks and would not have suggested psychotherapy, or who would have referred her to a psychologist or a social worker if she wanted to discuss her relationship with her parents. There is a great deal of ambiguity in our field and some uncertainty about definitive treatment plans.

Who can benefit from psychotherapy? Clearly, to gain something from talk therapy, the patient needs to be able to talk, so patients with severe brain injuries or notable mental retardation are not usually offered treatment with insight-oriented psychotherapy. Patients with psychotic disorders who are unable to accurately assess reality are also not candidates for insight-oriented approaches. They usually do better with supportive therapy. Psychotherapy is not usually done at a time when someone's state of awareness is compromised, so people are not seen while they are intoxicated or physically ill. Some people know themselves and feel there is nothing to be gained from therapy—they say things like, "I don't believe in psychiatry." Just as we're not sure if someone's headache will be helped by aspirin until after she takes it, we're also not sure who can be helped by psychotherapy, and sometimes people are pleasantly surprised to find they can be helped by something they didn't believe in.

Dr. Linus treats patients with psychotherapy. He is good at it, loves getting to know his patients well, and finds it rewarding. He learned to do this type of treatment over the course of years, beginning in his residency training. All psychiatric training includes education about how to provide psychotherapy, but some training programs place more emphasis on this. Psychotherapy is a long process that develops over time, and there's not a great mechanism for students to watch it unwind. Most of the learning occurs without a live patient present. The student will see a patient and either audio record the sessions to play for an experienced supervisor or take very careful notes. The student then discusses the session, but psychotherapy supervisors do not usually meet the patient. The student's report may be skewed—just as a recounting of any conversation can be biased—and the supervisor can't always be sure the reporting is accurate. There is also mirror supervision, in which the supervisor watches the session through a one-way mirror. This is a terrific learning experience, but not every training institution has the necessary equipment and structure for it.

There is no way for a trainee to be a fly on the wall of an older, more seasoned psychotherapist over long periods. Even in the most ideal situation, when a trainee tapes patient sessions over time and is guided by a single supervisor from start to finish, or a supervisor observes the therapy sessions through a one-way mirror, the training still involves a relatively small number of patients.

It's difficult enough that there are a variety of patients, but there are also a variety of supervisory styles. Two supervisors may have very different perspectives on the same patient, and this can be confusing for a student therapist. It is one reason many residents-in-training will undergo their own psychotherapy as part of their education.

Psychiatrists are not required to undergo therapy unless they are specializing as psychoanalysts. Training programs vary in how strongly they encourage residents to consider their own personal psychotherapy, but many therapists see it as an essential part of the learning process. In some programs, therapy is viewed strictly as a treatment for illness, and no statements are issued about the benefits of an educational therapy.

Should psychiatrists undergo their own psychotherapy? We believe they should if they want to. Given the limited ways that students have to learn the skill, it can be very helpful to watch an older and more experienced therapist interact with a patient—in this case, oneself—and serve as a role model. The student therapist may gain insight into his own personal conflicts, especially those issues that may influence his work with patients down the road. Also, being a patient may provide valuable learning—to experience firsthand what it feels like to be vulnerable in such a relationship, and to experience the sense of feeling understood or misunderstood.

Many people who are drawn to being psychotherapists have an inquisitive nature. They like to look at patterns and relationships. They are curious about what makes humans act the way they do, and by extension, they are likely to be interested in their own motivations, reactions, and relationships. Furthermore, people who practice psychotherapy believe in its power; they feel there is value to articulating emotional life and to examining the internal world. Given this, a personal therapy may have some appeal, with or without the presence of a psychiatric disorder, and if the psychiatry resident wants to have a personal psychotherapy, he should. If he has a psychiatric illness, he should certainly get treatment. But a psychiatry resident who is not ill, who is not suffering emotionally, and who does not want to have psychotherapy should not feel compelled to do so for its own sake. If he later decides it might be helpful to his work, there's no time limit—it's not just for trainees.

When Tara Jackson sought treatment, she was having terrible panic attacks. She would wake up in the middle of the night because her heart was pounding, and she had this horrible sense that she couldn't get enough air into her lungs. Sometimes the panic came on during the day, and she was terrified it would happen when she was driving. By the time she saw Dr. Linus, she had stopped driving on highways. She was afraid she wouldn't be able to pull over to the shoulder in time. Tara lived in fear of these episodes. Her father told her she was spoiled—she'd had a good life and had no reason to be panicky—and he felt her decision to see a psychiatrist was self-indulgent. Her mother was kind about listening but had nothing helpful to offer.

"I had a panic attack last night," Tara told Dr. Linus. "It's been happening a lot lately."

"What brought it on?" Dr. Linus asked.

"Nothing," Tara answered. She looked a bit exasperated. "They were better for a long time there. But I come each week, and it feels like we've talked about what triggers my panic attacks a zillion times. I feel like I've told you about everything that's ever happened in my life, and I should have this worked through by now. All this therapy, and I'm still having panic attacks. I know, you're going to suggest I do something different with the medicine, but I thought by now I wouldn't need pills anymore."

"You're feeling frustrated that you're still having panic attacks," Dr. Linus said.

"Yes," Tara said.

"Do you think we should continue with therapy? You seem to say it's not helping."

"Oh, of course. Don't you think I should keep coming? It helps me to talk to you! I'd just like to know if I'll ever be 'cured.' "

Dr. Linus understood Tara's concern about her treatment. She was doing all the "right" things to get better—taking the medication as prescribed and working hard in therapy—yet she was still having symptoms. He wished he could guarantee her that the therapy would help, but the best he could do was tell her the likelihood of improvement for patients with panic disorder. He knew the research on the efficacy of psychotherapy for the condition (and in Tara's case, on the efficacy of psychotherapy in combination with medications), but he also knew the limitations of that research. Medications work well, and the therapy of choice for the panic symptoms is a targeted, cognitive-behavioral approach. In fact, Dr. Linus was working with the assumption that the medications were treating the panic symptoms—and Tara was right that he thought they needed some tweaking. The psychotherapy was targeting her life issues and relationships, not searching for a cure for her panic symptoms.

For a long time, psychiatrists assumed that psychotherapy was helpful for many conditions. We assumed this without rigorous studies and without asking very specific questions. Then, researchers began to ask questions in fairly specific ways. Is one type of psychotherapy better than another for treating a given diagnosis? Is therapy better than medications for treating that same illness, or does a combination work best? Research protocols now look at patients in terms of the severity of their symptoms before and after a specific type of treatment, and they treat psychotherapy as one variable, just like the addition of a medication. The questions are asked in much more precise ways than simply "Does it work?" We'll illustrate this by talking about how psychiatric research is conducted.

First, research subjects are sought who share the same psychiatric diagnosis. The problem must be measured with some type of scale, and often a structured interview is used to assess the severity of the illness. Note that patients are not screened for whether they find it helpful to articulate their feelings or whether they like to talk about themselves; the research question is whether a specific type of psychotherapy is effective for treating a specific diagnosis.

Once a research population is identified, the patients are divided into groups, and each group gets a different treatment. If the treatments include psychotherapy, then often a short-term therapy is used in which the people conducting the therapy have been trained in the same method. CBT lends itself to these short-term interventions. The research subjects are reassessed after the treatment is over. Studies like this allow us to make statements such as "Cognitive-behavioral therapy is an effective treatment for obsessive-compulsive disorder." The people who received this therapy showed more improvement than people who did not.

Longer-term, insight-oriented psychotherapies don't lend themselves to controlled research studies. It's difficult to train people to have uniform approaches to patients, and it's difficult to fund research for long-term treatments. This doesn't mean that research is not possible; it just means it's not feasible to get a group of people with the same diagnosis and have one group see psychoanalysts for five years while the other group does not, and then assess if the treatment group gets better! What is more realistic is to do a retrospective, after-the-fact survey of patients who have been in long-term treatments to find out if they felt that treatment helped. These studies have value, but they don't have the scientific rigor and validity of studies in which the research subjects are chosen, measured for their symptoms, randomly assigned to treatment regimens, and then measured again to see if the treatments were effective. And finally, because the therapeutic relationship often provides solace, people will frequently identify treatment as being helpful even if their symptoms don't get better.

Tara knew the difference between feeling better and getting better. Even though she still had symptoms, she found it helpful to have a therapist who was genuine, warm, and empathetic to her problems. Early in treatment, Dr. Linus taught her about her illness, her symptoms, and her medications. Support and education are often the early goals of therapy. The long-term goal of therapy depends on the patient's reason for seeking treatment and how easily the patient can articulate her reflections on life.

Just as psychiatrists have different styles, patients also have different styles. Some like to talk about their lives by reporting every detail. Others come to a session and announce that "nothing" has happened since their last appointment. Patients may or may not talk about their lives in a way that moves toward their treatment goals. People often simply talk about the events of their week: what movies they saw, what parties they went to, or who said what in a disagreement. Patients may spend time talking about their home improvements, issues with their children, computers that crash, cars that need repair, books they've read, or events they've attended. These topics may sound superficial, but they are the fabric of people's lives. Therapy is often about the day-to-day events that an individual deals with. The psychotherapist's training and the patient's inclination to examine these different areas affect which issues the two of them will explore. Some people come very frequently and talk openly but make few changes. Others come rarely and get a great deal out of every session. Some psychiatrists give patients fairly specific instructions about what they should talk about, a process called *role induction*.

Tara didn't need much help when she started therapy. She talked about her life with a he said–she said detail that made Dr. Linus feel like he was in the room with Tara and her parents. Sometimes she simply gave a general interpretation.

"My mother uses me to make herself feel good," she said.

"Can you give me an example?" Dr. Linus asked. He might reach the same conclusion, but he wanted to get there himself.

Dr. Linus listened intently, which is crucial to good treatment. Often, he asked for more detail, or found something telling and guided the conversation down a certain path. Sometimes, he was there to offer hope and reassurance, especially when Tara's panic attacks were incapacitating or her relationships were in turmoil.

Psychotherapy is often about finding and elucidating patterns for people. *Have you noticed you always feel bad at this time of year? That you've been feeling worse since we stopped the medicine? How you talk about your boss the same way you talk about your mother? How you make assumptions about the reactions of strangers that keep you from even trying to get what you want?*

Dr. Linus helped Tara to see how her father kept her dependent and didn't nurture her growth as a competent adult. He also helped her to see her own role in allowing this to continue. Finally, he helped her to realize that her father was not all bad, that he loved her and had tried to be a good parent, and that he wanted to have a relationship with her. Her father had had a rough life, had worked hard, and though he wasn't perfect, he was not an evil man. Tara might alter the dynamic of her relationship with her father, but Dr. Linus helped her to accept that she wasn't going to change him.

Sometimes psychotherapy is about helping a patient to change. Other times, it is about helping a patient to accept who he is with less self-criticism and angst. Often it's about getting people to recognize their strengths and capitalize on them, rather than focusing so heavily on their weaknesses.

"I keep messing up at work," Tara said.

"Really?"

"I was late to a meeting on Friday, and I didn't get a report out on time."

"Did this upset your boss?"

"No, he was later than I was, and he asked me about the report, but by then I'd finished it."

"So how do you keep messing up?" Dr. Linus asked.

"I should have been on time to the meeting, and I should have finished the report early."

"That's funny. I don't hear that you're messing up. You sound like a very competent employee—in fact, you mentioned a few weeks ago that you'd gotten an excellent review and a raise. Perhaps you're hard on yourself? Maybe you hold yourself to an unreasonably high standard?"

Psychotherapy can involve pointing out things that would be difficult, painful, or insulting to hear in an ordinary conversation. The setting makes it safe to hear criticism and to learn about oneself in a way that enables change. How well the patient takes it depends on the skill of the psychotherapist; no one wants their faults shouted at them, and people hear these things best when their flaws aren't presented in harsh terms.

Another way of making observations is to examine the relationship between the patient and the psychiatrist, a technique that is common in insight-oriented psychotherapy. The concept of *transference* refers to the idea that the therapeutic relationship may involve the repetition of feelings the patient has had for other people, often parents or authority figures from childhood. It's a concept that comes from psychoanalytic theory, and not all psychiatrists believe it's important to fully examine these feelings.

"You're running late," Tara said when Dr. Linus didn't appear until ten minutes after one. She used her lunch hour to come to treatment, and she was clearly annoyed that she'd had to wait.

"You're displeased," he said. "I'm sorry that I'm late. I had an emergency this morning, and once I get behind, my whole day gets a little backed up."

Dr. Linus explained his behavior with the assumption that Tara's feelings reflected a realistic issue in their relationship. He might have chosen not to apologize and to explore her anger. In that case, the session would have included a different dialogue.

"How do you feel about my being late?" Dr. Linus might ask.

"Annoyed. You know I'm pressed for time."

"It feels like I'm not very respectful of that?"

"Well, yes," Tara might say.

"Perhaps it feels a little like when your father is dismissive of the responsibilities you have?"

Dr. Linus, however, did not choose that path. He knew he was running late, and he knew they were addressing Tara's issues with her father successfully without looking at her feelings about her doctor. He chose, instead, to address the issue of his own lateness and her discomfort with it on a face-value level.

Tara Jackson continued in therapy with Philip Linus. They talked about her life and her problems. He offered little about himself. He didn't wear a wedding ring or have any family photos on display in his office. She wondered if he even had a family. Tara assumed Dr. Linus was from Alabama because he had the remnants of a southern accent, and the diploma on the wall was from the University of Alabama. She knew he played the saxophone because she found some of his music on the Internet, and she knew he once owned a golden retriever who had died, because he had volunteered this information when she talked about how painful her own dog's death was.

While discussing the death of her dog, Tara had been surprised and a little disconcerted to learn that her veterinarian, Dr. Wright, was Dr. Linus's next-door neighbor. She found herself wondering if Dr. Linus and the vet ever discussed their patients, and if her case might be a topic of neighborhood dinner party conversation. Finally, she brought the issue up in therapy:

"Do you talk to Dr. Wright about me?" Tara asked.

Dr. Linus smiled. "No. I don't repeat anything you say." He reassured her that her treatment was confidential and that he could not tell Dr. Wright that she was his patient.

Privacy and confidentiality are keystones to psychiatric treatment. Patients tell doctors information that is personal and sometimes embarrassing. No one would do this if they couldn't trust the doctor to keep a secret. Patients may wonder if doctors can really do this. After all, doctors are human.

This is what the American Medical Association's Code of Medical Ethics says about the importance of medical secrets:

> The information disclosed to a physician by a patient should be held in confidence. The patient should feel free to make a full disclosure of information to the physician in order that the physician may most effectively provide needed services. The patient should be able to make this disclosure with the knowledge that the physician will respect the confidential nature of the communication. The physician should not reveal confidential information without the express consent of the patient, subject to certain exceptions which are ethically justified because of overriding considerations.

What are those "certain exceptions," and what kind of "overriding considerations" would allow a doctor to reveal information without permission? Both state and federal laws mandate medical confidentiality, but these laws also allow for disclosure of information if certain conditions are met. In some cases, the laws actually require doctors to report information. Typically this only occurs when there is an urgent need to protect someone—either the patient himself or the general public. Then doctors can (or must) reveal information to the police or to public health officials, such as the patient's name, address, phone number or other contact information, and the reason the doctor thinks the patient might be dangerous. All states have laws requiring psychiatrists to protect or notify intended victims of violent patients, and this necessitates a breach of confidentiality. All states also have laws requiring doctors to report child abuse.

Laws allow disclosure without written notice in order to investigate Medicaid or insurance fraud, or upon receipt of a valid subpoena or court order. When there is an allegation of malpractice or patient abuse, state laws allow disclosure of patient records to regulatory or licensure boards. A typical hospital consent for treatment form contains a provision requiring the patient to allow disclosure for the purposes of quality-assurance and utilization review. What does that mean? Aggregate information—in other words, information that is grouped together among patients and stripped of identifying data—is used for health care administration and medical research.

People sometimes get confused about the difference between confidentiality and testimonial privilege. *Testimonial privilege* refers to the patient's right to keep her doctor from testifying about confidential information. The issue of privilege only comes up when the medical information is needed for a legal proceeding. In most jurisdictions, there is no testimonial privilege if the patient makes his mental state an issue in a civil or criminal case. For example, if a patient files a civil suit and alleges that she suffered a psychological injury from someone's negligence, the defense would be able to get the plaintiff-patient's records and even require the doctor to testify. Similarly, a criminal defendant who files an insanity plea would not be able to keep his records secret.

The evolution of information technology has created new ways for medical information to be stored—and potentially breached. The Health Information and Portability Accountability Act (HIPAA) is a federal law that regulates how doctors, hospitals, and insurance companies protect the privacy of sensitive health information. HIPAA also sets encryption and storage standards for the security of electronic health information. Any doctor covered by HIPAA must abide by these regulations.

Verbal communications are also restricted by confidentiality laws. Typically a doctor will ask the patient's permission to discuss a case with a colleague as a consultation. On an inpatient unit, however, permission is not required to discuss a case within the treatment team. The unit nurses, doctors, psychologists, social workers, occupational therapists, and others consulting on the case are considered to be within the "circle of trust" and are not required to get consent for discussion. Other forms of verbal communication include presentations at educational conferences or internal case presentations, and all identifying information is usually removed from the case.

For court-ordered evaluations, such as child custody or visitation evaluations, it is possible to obtain medical records without patient consent. Although one could legally challenge the need for this information, records are rarely excluded from these cases because of their pertinence to the legal issue. In this case, the information and the generated report belong to the agency who ordered the evaluation. The court-ordered report belongs to the judge who requested it or to the retaining attorney, not to the patient.

Patients are notified about their privacy rights and informed about how their treatment information will be used during the informed consent process. At hospitals and clinics, patients are given privacy notices along with their informed consent documents. They are often asked to sign waivers as a condition of treatment that allow doctors to share information with insurance companies, those responsible for hospital quality-assurance or utilization-review processes, and others involved in managing health care systems. Psychiatrists who work for employee assistance programs or student mental health clinics may be expected to share information about the patient's need for workplace accommodation, fitness for duty, or potential for violence. In the case of employee assistance programs, the Americans With Disabilities Act requires employers to safeguard medical information and to disclose it only to managers or supervisors who need to provide accommodation.

The Patriot Act adopted in 2001 allows federal security investigators to obtain medical records without the consent or knowledge of the patient. This is done through a document called a national security letter. A doctor who receives a national security letter is forbidden from informing the patient that the information was requested, and those who do so face criminal penalties. Security letters can be issued if disclosure of the information is related to matters of national importance.

Besides protecting privacy, medical confidentiality laws ensure that patients have access to their own information as well as a means to correct inaccurate information. Medical records can be released directly to the patient upon receipt of a written request. In some states, there is a criminal penalty or fine for failing to release records. The data and information contained in the record belong to the patient, but the physical record itself belongs to the physician. Doctors can charge fees for copying time and cost. If the whole record isn't required, doctors may instead offer to write a letter documenting the diagnosis, any remaining symptoms, and the course of treatment to date.

These laws and acts don't become issues for the average psychiatrist on an average day. Most psychiatrists won't have encounters that are covered under the Patriot Act! None of this was related to Tara's care or to her concern that Dr. Linus might talk to Dr. Wright about her, and Tara was reassured that her information was safe with Dr. Linus, and that he wouldn't be repeating anything without her permission.

"I didn't know you were neighbors," Tara said. "You don't usually tell me about your life."

"No, I don't. Therapy is about you, and I don't want us to get diverted. I did want you to know that Dr. Wright is a wonderful vet, and that I think you did your best by Fido."

Tara was silent for a moment. "Sometimes I wonder what your life is like," she said.

While confidentiality refers to information that is kept secret by the doctor, the term *self-disclosure* refers to the doctor telling the patient information about himself. It may include details of his professional life, such as where he studied and his research interests. It may include more personal information that comes up in the course of conversation, such as a book he's read, a movie he's seen, what baseball team he roots for, or that his next-door neighbor is the patient's veterinarian.

The psychiatrist may, however, become more detailed and personal, telling a patient information about his family, or where he's gone on vacation. We talk about this more in a later chapter, where we discuss boundaries in psychotherapy. Because patients in psychotherapy talk about the intimate details of their own lives, the psychiatrist may feel it is helpful to share specific facts about his own life at select moments. Sometimes it helps the patient to feel understood, such as by sharing the sadness over the death of a dog, and sometimes it entails just being a kind human being, such as sharing the joy in homemade cookies over the holidays.

One of the features of any type of medical treatment, however, is that the treatment is about the patient. In an appointment with a dentist, or a primary care doctor, it may be fine for the doctor to tell an interested patient about his life—what his wife does, where he's traveled—or to converse about issues he and the patient have in common. Even in those settings, it's important that the appointment be focused on addressing the patient's concerns. It's nice if both the doctor and patient enjoy their discussion about a political candidate or a football trade, but not if the patient leaves before his chest pain was addressed.

The unidirectional flow of information is one of the boundaries that differentiates psychotherapy from friendship. Self-disclosure in psychotherapy gets particular scrutiny because of psychotherapy's underpinnings in Freudian psychoanalytic theory, in which the therapist is required to be a blank slate. For this type of treatment to work, the patient knows as little as possible about the therapist's personal life. The patient's curiosity about the doctor may yield some insights, and the patient is free to project her own ideas or fantasies onto the psychoanalyst. Here, self-disclosure isn't just imprudent, it's actually considered to be harmful to the treatment. From this, we've gotten all those jokes about how psychiatrists answer a question with a question!

Self-disclosure may occur spontaneously or at the request of the patient. Perhaps a patient wants to relay how something she saw in a movie resonated with her. She starts a lengthy description of the plot and characters, and the psychiatrist tells her he has seen the movie. This enables the patient to skip the background details and jump right to the part of the plot she wished to share. Another psychiatrist may choose to withhold the fact that he's seen the movie.

Sometimes patients feel a particular need to know something specific about their psychiatrist and may ask personal questions. Perhaps it's something the patient wants to know in order to relate to the doctor, such as his religious or cultural background. In these cases, the doctor must decide what he is comfortable disclosing. One major reason a physician may choose not to answer personal questions is because he wants, and is entitled to, his privacy.

That said, the reality is that no one is a totally blank slate, and no one gets complete privacy. Sometimes it's only reasonable to tell patients about a medical condition the therapist is coping with. It's difficult to hide a pregnancy, and perhaps patients are entitled to know if their therapists are anticipating a prolonged leave.

What about a situation in which the psychiatrist has a psychiatric disorder himself? There is nothing inherently wrong, immoral, or illegal about a therapist telling a patient that he suffers from a psychiatric disorder. If the therapist doesn't mind the loss of privacy and doesn't then use the sessions to talk about his own problems, it's not wrong, but it can be powerful, so there are possible risks and benefits.

As in any conversation, whether something said is helpful or harmful is subject to Monday morning quarterbacking and interpretation, and we don't always control how information is taken or used. A patient can have many responses, including the thought that it's troubling to know the therapist has a mental illness. She may feel burdened by the therapist's problems. If the patient is distressed by a therapist's self-disclosure, then it was the wrong thing to do. If the patient is comforted by their shared condition (especially when the doctor can offer hope and a good outcome), then it was the right thing to do.

When people are diagnosed with a brain tumor, they want a neurosurgeon with wonderful technical skills who has had success in treating tumors like theirs. They want the best surgeon, not the nicest person, and generally, people with serious illnesses don't care about their surgeon's background. When people look for a psychiatrist, they sometimes care about very specific personal characteristics. It's not at all unusual for people to specifically request a female psychiatrist. And while patients are not usually particular about the personal lives of a psychiatrist they see for medication management, they sometimes express a desire to see a psychotherapist with certain characteristics. Patients may want to see someone who shares their racial, religious, or ethnic background; they may want someone who speaks their native language; or they may want to talk to someone with the same sexual orientation. This is one reason that patients might ask a psychiatrist to disclose personal information. Sometimes this happens over the phone before the two parties even meet.

Does it help to have a therapist who is familiar in some ways with the patient's world or culture or core beliefs? Just as some patients respond to one medication and not another, some people have very strong feelings about who they are comfortable speaking with, while others don't care. For psychotherapy, it may matter.

Many people live in areas with limited access to psychiatric care, and choice is not an option. In an ideal world, anything reasonable that makes a patient more comfortable should be accommodated as long as it doesn't make someone else uncomfortable.

Dr. Linus gave Tara a medication when she first consulted him, and her symptoms resolved within a few weeks. Her panic attacks were cured— or so she believed. When they briefly returned, Dr. Linus adjusted the dose of medication, and Tara was able to identify some of the things that had precipitated her panic attacks. She was better, but she still met with Dr. Linus regularly for psychotherapy after her acute symptoms were treated.

Tara came because she was having panic attacks, and in the course of talking, she realized that her relationship with her parents was affecting her life negatively, and she wanted to continue to work on this in weekly therapy sessions. As time went by, she sorted through some of her issues, and eventually she bought a condominium and moved out of her parents' home. As much as her father objected to this, the separation helped their relationship. Tara saw Dr. Linus for weekly sessions for fourteen months. As she got better, other things seemed to take priority, and she wanted to come less often. For another six months, she went every other week, then monthly. She took medications for panic disorder for almost three years. After she went off the medications, Tara told Dr. Linus she wanted to call him to schedule the next session; she called three months later. From there on, she saw Dr. Linus a few times a year, and she continued to find their sessions helpful. At one point, after her second child was born, Tara was having a rough time, and they scheduled more frequent sessions. All told, Tara saw Dr. Linus for twelve years, until he moved out of state.

Twelve years may sound like a long time to be in treatment, but there is no definitive answer to the question of how long treatment should last. Doctors deal with this question on a case-by-case basis. Many illnesses are lifelong conditions that require varying degrees of intervention, so the answer is an individual and a personal one. It makes sense to stop and evaluate every few months whether things are getting better. Is there another way to go at the problem, or is there something more, or different, that can be done? If the answer is repeatedly "No change at all," then it's reasonable to get another opinion or try something completely different.

Many patients have chronic, repeated, or treatment-resistant forms of mental illness, and if they are seen frequently, it is easier to catch an episode and intervene early. Regular therapy sessions may keep them grounded and prevent recurrence. In these cases, therapy has been referred to as a holding environment.

In a traditional psychoanalysis, the termination of therapy is planned well in advance. Ideally, in any insight-oriented psychotherapy, the ending would be a planned event. More often, patients either taper the frequency of sessions and then stop coming, or they come for a regularly scheduled appointment and say that they'd like this to be their final session because they feel better. Ideally, it should be the patient who decides when the work is done or when it no longer feels necessary or useful.

Ultimately, psychotherapy is about what the patient wants and her perception of what is helpful. Sometimes therapy is about minimizing distress; other times, it's about maximizing what someone gets out of life; and sometimes it is about preventing relapse and maintaining a status quo.

Chapter 5

Josh Revisited:
"Ask Your Doctor to Prescribe"

REMEMBER JOSH from chapter 2? In the course of his illness, Josh was treated with several psychiatric medications, so we're going to revisit him while we talk about how medications are used in psychiatry. In this chapter, we talk about how psychiatrists choose medications, and what they do when patients don't get better right away. We talk about the patient's right to know about the risks of medications and procedures, a process called informed consent. With some medications, for example, there is a risk of addiction, and this presents a particular challenge to psychiatrists. Finally, we talk about treatment-resistant conditions and a little about what the future might hold as we strive for better ways to help patients.

Josh first saw Dr. Smith because he was depressed, and Dr. Smith clarified that Josh was suffering from a mental illness. His symptoms were not simply manifestations of adolescent angst, trouble adjusting to college, or stress. Dr. Smith recommended both medication and psychotherapy for Josh's depression.

You'll remember that Josh had a rather complicated story. He became depressed and was treated with an antidepressant. This medication quickly caused him to become hypomanic, that is, his mood and energy level were elevated too far above the normal, a process known as *switching*. Josh was then taken off the antidepressant and given a mood stabilizer, and for quite some time, he did well, but then an unfortunate series of events transpired. Josh played soccer in the cold, got the flu, and went into a smoke-filled room, and all these things triggered a terrible asthma attack. Josh needed to take steroids for his asthma, and this medication induced a full-blown episode of mania during which Josh became psychotic and dangerous and was admitted involuntarily to a psychiatric hospital, where he was treated with even more medications.

In this chapter, we borrow Josh to explain the issues a psychiatrist thinks about when prescribing psychotropic medications.

When doctors think about medications, they usually think in terms of the illness that the medication treats. For example, antineoplastic drugs treat cancer, and antibiotic medications treat infections. Psychiatric medications are a little different. They are grouped by the symptoms they target. There are antidepressants to treat depression, mood stabilizers to treat and prevent mania, antianxiety agents and sedative-hypnotics to help with anxiety and sleep, and antipsychotic medications to target hallucinations and delusions and prevent relapses of schizophrenia. The medication classifications, however, don't work very well for describing their uses. For example, antidepressants treat depression, but they are also commonly prescribed to treat anxiety disorders. Mood-stabilizing medications are used to treat and prevent mania, but they are also used to augment, or boost, the actions of other medications in the treatment of depression. Antipsychotic medications target hallucinations and delusions and prevent relapses of the acute symptoms of schizophrenia, but they may also be used to help with mood stabilization and agitation even if a patient is not psychotic. Sometimes low doses of antipsychotic medicines are prescribed for depression and sleep problems. In these cases, the medicine is being used for an off-label purpose, which means the Food and Drug Administration has determined the medication's safety, but efficacy has not been proven for that specific condition. When the approved medicines don't work or cannot be used, physicians will often prescribe medications off-label. Psychotropic medications may be prescribed for a number of conditions, so the drug classifications are often misleading indicators of what they are treating.

Josh was depressed, and he started taking an antidepressant. There are many different antidepressants, including Prozac, Paxil, Zoloft, Lexapro, Celexa, Luvox, Effexor, Cymbalta, Pristiq, Wellbutrin, Remeron, Serzone,

Pamelor, Elavil, Nardil, Parnate, Emsam, Desyrel, and Sinequan. With so many medications to choose from, how did Josh's psychiatrist, Dr. Smith, know which one to try?

Dr. Smith considered many things when he chose a medication for Josh. First, he decided what class of medications to use—in Josh's case, an antidepressant—and from there, he considered several factors:

Past History of Response. If Josh had said, "Oh, yeah, six years ago I felt this way, and I took Paxil. It helped a lot, and I didn't have any side effects," then Dr. Smith would have prescribed Paxil. If Josh had tried medications that didn't work or had side effects, Dr. Smith would have avoided prescribing those drugs for him. But Josh had never been on any psychotropic medication, so there were many possible options.

Family History of Response. What if Josh's mother had said that Wellbutrin was the only antidepressant that had ever worked for her? Genes certainly have a role in susceptibility to mental disorders, and they may well have a role in determining response to medications. If Wellbutrin helped a family member, it might help Josh. No one in Josh's family was taking an antidepressant, although his mother was taking Depakote for her bipolar disorder.

Patient Preference. Another patient said his best friend took Celexa and got much better. He didn't know what the friend's diagnosis was or why Celexa was chosen, but the patient wanted to try that particular medication. If there wasn't a contraindication, or the psychiatrist didn't feel strongly that another medication was a better choice, then he would prescribe the medication the patient requested. Dr. Smith felt there was power in the belief that a medication might help. Similarly, if the patient reported that Celexa caused his best friend to have awful side effects and that he wanted any medication *but* Celexa, then the psychiatrist would prescribe something else. Josh did not come to treatment with any specific requests about medications.

Other Medications. Medications can interact with each other in dangerous and even life-threatening ways. Dr. Smith asked Josh what medications he was taking. Josh had just started something new for his asthma, but he couldn't remember the name. Dr. Smith called Josh's pharmacy and got the name of the medication, then checked for drug interactions.

He didn't want to prescribe anything that would be dangerous in conjunction with Josh's other medications. There were not any common antidepressants that couldn't be prescribed with Josh's asthma medications.

Best Guess as to What Will Help the Target Symptoms. Josh was tired and unmotivated, so Wellbutrin might have been a good choice for him because it increases energy and motivation in some patients. Remeron causes weight gain and promotes sleep in some people, so it is a good choice for a patient who suffers from poor appetite and insomnia. It's not ideal for a patient who is overweight and is sleeping too much.

Co-morbid Conditions. Sometimes it's possible to address two problems with one medication. For example, some antidepressants also treat obsessive-compulsive disorder; others also treat pain syndromes. Josh had mentioned that his teachers thought he had attentional problems when he was young. Wellbutrin can be used as a treatment for attention deficit disorder, and if Josh had still been having attention problems (he hadn't been), then this might have been one more reason to use it.

Best Guess at the Side-Effect Profile. This is very much a guess—few medications induce a specific side effect in every patient who takes them. Aspirin causes upset stomachs, but certainly not in everyone, so while it should be avoided in a patient with a known history of bleeding ulcers, it will not necessarily cause gastrointestinal problems in someone who isn't predisposed. Predicting side effects is really a matter of odds. We know which medicines have a high likelihood, and which have a low likelihood, of causing problems. Dr. Smith did not want to choose a medication that was likely to further suppress Josh's appetite, and Wellbutrin might have done that. He decided not to prescribe a tricyclic antidepressant, such as Elavil, because it was more likely to cause dry mouth and fatigue. Even though there were several reasons to try Wellbutrin, Dr. Smith was very concerned about Josh's weight loss, and he prescribed a selective serotonin reuptake inhibitor (SSRI) called Zoloft, or sertraline. He warned Josh that it could interfere with his sex drive and told him to let him know if this happened.

Concerns about Long-Term Consequences of the Medication. Some medications are associated with problems over time. The older antipsychotic medications, known as neuroleptics, can cause irreversible movement disorders. The newer antipsychotic agents can cause changes in metabolism that contribute to obesity, diabetes, and lipid abnormalities. Lithium, a mood stabilizer, can affect a patient's kidney or thyroid function. And many antianxiety medications can result in dependence and addiction. Often the patient's acute need for treatment will overwhelm the concern about longer-term consequences, but these issues will eventually need to be addressed if a patient remains on a medication.

Financial Concerns. Some patients want the medication with the best efficacy and side-effect profile regardless of the price. Others request a cheaper medication. Insurance companies may have formularies that do not include certain medications, or that require patients to pay more for them. Sometimes the choice of medication is based on what free samples the physician has available, so the patient can at least try the drug at no cost. Medications can be very expensive, and cost may be a major factor.

The Doctor's Past Experience with That Particular Medication. Often, doctors like certain medicines because their patients have gotten better with them before. Other times, a doctor has seen a problem with a medication and does not want to prescribe it again. These issues are not always about evidence-based studies and may reflect the emotional and anecdotal experiences of the doctor. This is true in all fields of medicine, not just psychiatry. Doctors have favorite medications. Dr. Smith had prescribed Zoloft many times before. Most patients tolerated it well, and many found it to be helpful. It was often his first choice medication for depression.

Outside Influences. We like to believe that physicians choose medications with only the best interest of their patients in mind, but physicians are often pressured in many ways. Insurance companies may require that they fill out forms and get preauthorization to prescribe certain medications, and this extra step certainly deters doctors from using these medications when it is easier to prescribe something else. Pharmaceutical companies influence physicians through enticements and free samples of medications. Physicians may have concerns about how our resources are used as a society and may feel it is socially more responsible to try a less expensive medication first, even if the possibility of side effects is higher.

Zoloft was actually not the right medicine for Josh. In just a few days, his depression was better, but he felt "too good." The medications that are used to treat mental illnesses have risks associated with them, and the decision to take those risks or not can be a difficult one. Because Josh had a family history of bipolar disorder, Dr. Smith warned him that he might become manic. Josh also became manic when he took steroids for his asthma, but that episode was much, much worse. These reactions might have indicated that Josh had bipolar disorder, but because his episodes were both induced by medications, Dr. Smith could not say for sure if Josh would need medications to treat bipolar disorder forever. He thought it was likely.

Because patient preference plays a role in the doctor's decision to prescribe a certain medication, regardless of what is chosen, patients need to consider a lot of information before they decide whether to take a given medication. This isn't always easy to do. Lack of energy, difficulty with concentration or memory, and feelings of hopelessness or worthlessness can hinder a patient's decision-making abilities.

Nevertheless, the patient has a right to know what treatments are available, how likely they are to help, and what the risks of those treatments are. The process by which a doctor disseminates this information is known as informed consent. Josh was prescribed an antidepressant and then a mood stabilizer as an outpatient, and he was informed of the risks. Later, when he became manic after he took the steroids for his asthma, he was committed to the psychiatric unit, and he was treated with intramuscular injections of sedatives as well as oral doses of a mood stabilizer and an antipsychotic agent. The risks of the medications were explained to him, and he was told about some of the side effects that might occur. If Josh had chosen not to take medications, he would have been told the risks and benefits of that choice. During an emergency, a doctor is not legally required to give informed consent to begin treatment.

Psychiatrists and other physicians take the process of informed consent for granted today, but medicine wasn't always that way. As recently as the 1960s, the standard of practice in medicine was for a physician to tell the patient only what the doctor thought the patient needed to know. This viewpoint, or practice, was called the *reasonable physician standard*. In other words, the type or amount of information given to the patient was based on what a reasonable doctor, using ordinary care, would give to a patient.

The reasonable physician standard of informed consent eventually gave way to the *material risk standard,* in 1972. In the legal case *Canterbury v. Spence,* a 19-year-old patient named Jerry Canterbury underwent spinal surgery to correct back pain. His doctor told his mother that the operation was no more serious than any other surgery and neglected to mention a remote possibility of paralysis from the procedure. When Canterbury eventually did experience paralysis, he sued the surgeon, alleging that the doctor had not enabled him to give informed consent. The doctor argued that warning a patient about every possible bad outcome could deter patients from seeking needed care and could even cause psychological harm. The United States Court of Appeals disagreed and said that it was the physician's duty to disclose any material risk. A material risk meant any potential harm from the treatment that was either frequent enough or serious enough to influence a reasonable patient to either accept or refuse the treatment.

Psychiatric patients have a right to know the material risks of psychiatric care. In general, this refers to the risks associated with psychiatric medications. The amount of information given about a specific medication will depend on the drug that's being prescribed and how much is known about it. With medications that have been around for years, like lithium (a mood-stabilizing medication), the risks are well known and easy to list. For newer medications, the risks may not all be known yet. Unfortunately, there can sometimes be very serious risks associated with new medications that aren't discovered during the drug approval process. When the weight loss drugs fenfluramine and phentermine (fen-phen) were prescribed for dieters, doctors didn't know that fenfluramine carried an increased risk of causing leaky heart valves. Fenfluramine was eventually pulled from the market and is no longer available. The older antipsychotic medications can cause a movement disorder called tardive dyskinesia. This did not become apparent until many years after psychiatrists began prescribing these medications, because this disorder occurs only after years of exposure to the drugs.

Informed consent is easier for patients now because so much information is available through the Internet, but it's important to find accurate sources of information. Both the National Institute of Mental Health and the Food and Drug Administration provide information for patients about psychiatric medications. Several sites also provide patient educational materials or medical literature searches. Pharmacies typically provide information about medications when they dispense prescriptions.

Doctors don't usually answer questions by quoting statistics. There are a lot of medications out there, and the entire list of side effects for any one medication can be quite long. Statistics about risk are not something a doctor is able to carry around in her head, but it is possible to break down risks into general categories of "common," "occasional," and "almost never but potentially serious so you should know about it." Finally, despite all good pharmaceutical research, sometimes weird things happen. There's always that one patient who has the misfortune of being the first reported case of a serious reaction, and doctors don't have any way of predicting that. Patients sometimes get angry when a medication causes them more harm than good, and they sometimes feel the doctor should have warned them, or should not have prescribed that medication. The truth is that there is risk involved whenever someone takes a pill or has a procedure. When a patient is having disruptive and disabling symptoms and does not want to even try a medication because of the fear of side effects (that might not happen), or the fear of a bad reaction, it can be very difficult for everyone involved. Patients have the right to refuse medications, but sometimes doctors and family wish they'd give them a try because of the chance they might help a great deal.

"Janine says the medicines are the problem. She thinks I should try St. John's Wort or supplements," Josh told Dr. Smith.

Janine was Josh's stepsister. She ate a strict vegan diet and felt that good nutrition held more promise for Josh than conventional medicine. She blamed his symptoms on the medications, but Dr. Smith pointed out to Josh that he had been suffering from a severe and debilitating depressive episode before he'd ever tried a medication.

Some patients prefer to try alternative medications and supplements, which we talk about in more detail in chapter 11. Some examples of supplements used to address mood disorders include St. John's Wort, fish oil supplements, and SAM-e (S-adensyl methionine). Some nutritional supplements may have therapeutic value. Omega-3 fatty acids, specifically eicosapentaenoic acid (ECA) and docosahexaenoic acid (DHA), have been studied for the treatment of depression and bipolar disorder. There are only a small number of studies using these fatty acids for a few months, but they suggest that ECA and DHA may cause short-term improvement in the course of bipolar disorder.

These therapies are not regulated by the Food and Drug Administration because they're nutritional supplements rather than medicines, and they have not been subject to the rigorous testing that medications must go through to determine their safety and efficacy. The National Center for the Study of Complementary and Alternative Medicine, a branch of the National Institutes of Health, researches safety and efficacy issues for some of these treatments, but they are still not regulated the way traditional medications are. There is now a reporting system to collect data about adverse reactions to alternative treatments and nutritional supplements. Some supplements are manufactured overseas where the manufacturing process isn't regulated, and we don't always know exactly what's in a given capsule. Ayurvedic preparations, herbal supplements imported from India, have been contaminated with heavy metals, and nutritional supplements have caused death from liver failure. Alternative and complementary treatments may work, but physicians often prefer treatment with medications that have been tested and regulated. Dr. Smith explained this to Josh and suggested they stick with traditional medications, at least for the moment.

During the course of his illness, Josh was on several medications at various doses. Psychiatrists usually start medications at low doses to minimize side effects. They gradually increase the dose as the patient gets used to it, which minimizes the risk of side effects. If a patient is very sick, the amount of medicine may be raised more quickly. The dose of a medication is raised until one of three things happens: the symptoms get better, intolerable side effects develop, or the maximum dose is reached. For antidepressants, it can take three to six weeks from the time the maximum dose is given until a response occurs. Some medications don't have an absolute maximum dose. Instead, the level of the medication is measured in the blood, and the dose is raised until the level is therapeutic. For Zoloft, the medication that Dr. Smith prescribed to Josh, the starting dose is 12.5 to 25 milligrams, and the maximum dose is 200 milligrams.

What if Josh got to the maximum dose of the medication and was no better at all? Dr. Smith would try another medicine. He might try another SSRI, or he might try a completely different class of antidepressants. He would again start at a low dose of the medicine and titrate up to a therapeutic dose.

What if Josh had gotten a little better on Zoloft, but not all the way better? Then, Dr. Smith would have had a few choices. If he'd thought it was safe, and if Josh had been having no side effects, he might have tried Josh on a dose that was above the usual maximum dose (off-label dosing). He would not do that if Josh had been on a medication known to be toxic at high doses. Another option would be to add a second medication, a strategy known as augmentation. He might augment the Zoloft with a second antidepressant from another class of medicines, or with a completely different type of medication, such as lithium or thyroid hormone.

What if this still didn't work? Dr. Smith could do the same thing again, adding a third medication. He could stop some of the medicines and try another class of medicine. If two medications fail after full trials at high enough doses, for long enough periods of time, then the patient has what is called *treatment-resistant depression*. It's important to note that it's the depression that is resisting treatment, not the patient.

The issues are similar with other conditions, such as mania and schizophrenia. Medications are given until a maximum dose is reached, assuming that the patient can tolerate the medicine. If that doesn't work, a new medicine is tried, or a second medicine is added. Sometimes patients are on two mood stabilizers. They are not usually on two antipsychotic medications of the same type. If several antipsychotic medications, tried one after another, don't work, and the patient continues to have hallucinations and delusions, he may be started on a medication called clozapine (Clozaril). This medication is associated with many serious side effects and the possibility of serious adverse effects, and it requires a great deal of monitoring, so it is a last resort medication for the treatment of schizophrenia. But it is an effective treatment and sometimes works when nothing else has helped.

What if nothing helped Josh? On rare occasions, nothing helps, and people stay very depressed for long periods. At that point, other treatments might be considered. Electroconvulsive therapy (ECT) is a powerful and effective treatment for depression, and it works in 90 percent of people. Patients are usually hospitalized for ECT the first time. They are given general anesthesia, and a seizure is induced. The patient is paralyzed by the anesthetic so that they can't hurt themselves during the seizure. ECT usually requires three treatments a week for six to twelve treatments. Side effects include headaches and memory loss, so ECT is reserved for serious cases of depression. We talk more about ECT in the chapter on hospital-based psychiatry.

Experimental procedures are available for treatment-resistant depression that has not responded to any of the usual therapies. Vagal nerve stimulation (VNS) involves surgically implanting a device in the chest beneath the collarbone to electrically stimulate the vagus nerve. In deep brain stimulation (DBS), an electrode is implanted in the brain so that current can be delivered directly to specific areas. For transcranial magnetic stimulation (TMS), the patient goes for daily hour-long visits and sits in a device that looks like a dentist's chair while the brain is magnetically stimulated. We don't know why any of these treatments work. They are expensive and time consuming, and they require special facilities. Still, they may offer relief to a select group of people when all else has failed.

Josh was not a candidate for any of these procedures because he got better within a few weeks. He continued to see Dr. Smith for therapy sessions, and he abstained from drinking alcohol and smoking marijuana.

Josh felt anxious one day after he got home from the hospital. His mother had some Xanax that her doctor had given her. She gave one to Josh, and it made him feel much better.

"Can I get a prescription for Xanax?" Josh asked Dr. Smith.

"Xanax?" Dr. Smith raised his eyebrows.

"My mom gave me one when I was upset, and it helped a lot."

"Just one?" Dr. Smith asked.

"Well, she gave me one. I helped myself to a few more," Josh said.

"Maybe not such a good idea," Dr. Smith said. He explained that Xanax was an addictive medication.

Controlled substances are medicines that carry a risk of dependence, abuse, or addiction. Pain medications, such as Oxycontin (extended-release oxycodone) or Percocet (a combination of oxycodone and acetaminophen), are in this category. Medications like Xanax (alprazolam), Valium (diazepam), Librium (chlordiazepoxide), Klonopin (clonazepam), and Ativan (lorazepam) are benzodiazepines, also called minor tranquilizers or sedatives. Benzodiazepines (often shortened to "benzos") may also become problematic, and psychiatrists sometimes avoid using medications that can lead to addiction for fear the cure will be worse than the disease. These medications are known as drugs of abuse, and sometimes prescriptions get diverted and sold on the street. Although Dr. Smith had no reason to believe that Josh wanted Xanax to sell, it's not at all uncommon for people to do this with addictive medications. Doctors who prescribe a lot of addictive medications may come under the scrutiny of the federal Drug Enforcement Agency, and they may be subject to professional, or even criminal, sanctions. Dr. Smith didn't think he'd get arrested if he gave Josh a few tablets of Xanax, but he knew Josh liked to binge drink and smoke marijuana, and he worried that Josh might have some predisposition toward addiction. He didn't think it was a good idea to expose him unnecessarily to this class of medications.

What is it about benzodiazepines that can make them so addictive? Some people have genetic factors that make them more or less prone to develop an addiction. Apart from such genetic predispositions, the addictive potential of this type of medication is also related to its pharmacologic half-life, potency, and fat solubility. The term half-life means the length of time it takes for a person's body to get rid of the medication. The half-life for alprazolam (Xanax) is short, on the order of six to twenty hours. Alprazolam is one of the most potent benzodiazepines. It is also quite *lipophilic*, meaning fat soluble, which is a big factor in how quickly a drug can get into the brain. Only diazepam (Valium) and chlorazepate (Tranxene) are more lipophilic than alprazolam. Since the brain is largely made of fat, lipophilic drugs will get into the brain more quickly. Thus, because of its high potency, short half-life, and lipophilicity, alprazolam gets into the brain quickly, does its thing, and then quickly goes away, so it has a quick-on, quick-off way of working. Almost like a switch. Sounds great, right?

When you have a cause-and-effect relationship, it becomes a stronger relationship when the effect occurs soon after the cause. The quicker a drug works, especially one that makes someone feel good in some way, the more addicting it can be. This is because the cause (taking it) and the effect (feeling it) are close in time, which makes it very reinforcing. This is not as much of a problem when someone needs a medication to get through those rare anxious moments—say, for extreme anxiety when flying. However, since alprazolam works so quickly, many folks start taking it more and more often, until they are taking it daily. Then they start taking another dose as soon as the last dose begins to wear off. Before they know it, they are taking it three to four times per day. Now, even *that's* not the big problem.

The big problem here is all because of the brain's laziness. The brain makes its own natural Xanax-like substance, called GABA, or gamma aminobutyric acid, that works by inhibiting the brain's natural tendency to send electrical impulses all over the place. GABA is like a brake pedal, keeping the brain's speed in check when the accelerator is stuck in the pedal-to-the-metal mode. GABA keeps the brain from working overtime. Alprazolam, as well as other sedatives and alcohol, works by acting like GABA in the brain. If someone takes it daily, the brain starts thinking, "I guess I don't need to make so much of my own GABA because this Xanax stuff is here, so I'll make only 20 percent of what I usually make." (Technically, it makes fewer GABA receptors, but the effect is the same for our discussion.) It takes a week or more for the brain to stop making the GABA, which is why just a few days on Xanax won't lead to much trouble, and it takes a week or more for it to start making it again when the patient stops taking the Xanax.

Here's where the trouble begins. If Xanax wears off in just a few hours, but it takes a week for the brain's natural Xanax to kick back in, what happens in the meantime? Withdrawal. What does that feel like? It feels like a panic attack, but worse. What do folks do when they feel a panic attack coming on? Take another Xanax. Benzodiazepine withdrawal, in its worst form, consists of high blood pressure, rapid heartbeat, tremors, confusion, delirium, hallucinations, and seizures. This withdrawal business can be dangerous stuff.

Older people may wind up with more severe withdrawal problems from stopping Xanax. They run out of the drug, decide to cut back, just stop taking it, or something else happens (for example, they have a stroke or get some other illness), and they forget to take it. Or they go into the hospital and don't tell their surgeon they are on it, so the doctor doesn't order any, and two days after their hip surgery, they start hallucinating from the delirium associated with acute Xanax withdrawal.

Withdrawal is one problem, addiction is another, and chronic use can lead to memory impairment, slower thinking, and slower reaction times. Older people who take benzodiazepines are also more susceptible to falls.

Some prescribers think that alprazolam is a good antidepressant (it's not). Or that because of the short half-life, it's not as addictive as other prescription medications (it is). Fortunately, most people can use alprazolam without problems of abuse or dependence.

Here are our rules of thumb about alprazolam. Like most rules of thumb, these are meant to be only a guide. Xanax is FDA approved for treating anxiety and panic disorder, and a blanket statement that Xanax should never be prescribed cannot be made.

- In general, avoid it.
- Keep the doses small.
- Avoid it in older folks and in people who are forgetful.
- Most people with a history of alcoholism or addiction should not be taking benzodiazepines or other addictive drugs.
- When taken daily, Xanax should not be stopped suddenly, even for a day or two, because doing so can result in severe withdrawal symptoms and delirium, including confusion, hallucinations, seizures, and rarely death. Patients can also have severe rebound anxiety, including panic attacks, when Xanax is stopped suddenly.

Dr. Smith talked with Josh about the dangers of Xanax. He told Josh he didn't think it would be in his best interest to continue taking it. Josh was fine with this, and they talked more about what made Josh anxious as well as about some nonpharmacologic ways he might address his uncomfortable feelings. Dr. Smith asked Josh to keep track of what made his anxiety better and what made it worse.

The use of benzodiazepines, even those with longer half-lives that aren't as addictive as Xanax or Valium, remains controversial in psychiatry. Most psychiatrists find them to be useful for short-term control of severe agitation, and many doctors prescribe them for events such as airplane flights or helping to remain relaxed during a stressful diagnostic test such as magnetic resonance imaging (MRI). The occasional or short-term use in a patient without an addiction is not generally a problem, as long as the medicine is not mixed with alcohol or narcotics. These medications can be extremely helpful for managing panic attacks and periodic anxiety.

Psychiatrists have different perspectives on the usefulness of benzodiazepines and sleep medications on a chronic basis, which we discuss in more detail in chapter 11. Some psychiatrists feel they are invaluable in the treatment of anxiety and insomnia and that taken as prescribed, they are safe and effective. Other psychiatrists feel that the risks of addiction and dependence outweigh the possible benefits, and that it can be very hard to tell if a patient wants to continue on the medication because it controls his symptoms in a helpful way or because a habit has developed.

Sometimes patients don't even realize they are addicted to the medications. When patients escalate the dose on their own, "lose" prescriptions or pills for controlled substances, or become very demanding about prescriptions, doctors worry that the patients have become addicted. These are behaviors we just don't see with medications that don't have this potential.

The choice of medications involves a degree of guesswork; we don't know who will respond to a medication, who will develop side effects, or who might be at risk for addiction to controlled substances. Will this always be the case?

A person's genes control how various substances, including medications, are metabolized by the body. Some people have multiple copies of the gene that breaks down a particular medication; those people metabolize that medication much more quickly, and the accumulated breakdown products, or metabolites, can cause side effects. The active medication also gets cleared from the body so quickly that it doesn't have time to work. These ultra-rapid metabolizers may not respond to the medication, but they still have trouble with side effects.

Other patients are missing the genes they need to metabolize a given medicine at a normal rate. It takes much longer for the drug to be cleared by the body. As a result, they are prone to toxicity from high levels of medication.

There are tests to determine how many copies of these genes a patient has, and we can tell if someone is a fast or slow metabolizer, but so many other factors are involved in medication response and in adverse reactions that we can't routinely predict outcomes. We hope to eventually understand all the factors, and we believe that someday, there may be ways of telling with a simple test who will respond to what drug. This is the promise of psychopharmacogenetics. Dr. Smith couldn't order a test that would predict that Josh would become manic on Zoloft, or which mood stabilizer was the right one for him, but in the future, that might change.

What ultimately happened to Josh? Did he do well? Was he successful?

Josh's college had several conditions for his return. Dr. Smith needed to verify that Josh was in treatment and that he was well enough to return to school. He was not allowed to return to the dorm. He stayed, instead, with an aunt and uncle and commuted to college from their house. He was seen by a therapist at the school counseling center, and he returned home every other week for a Friday afternoon appointment with Dr. Smith.

Josh eventually had another manic episode, one that was not precipitated by a medication, and it became clear that he did have bipolar disorder. Some people with bipolar disorder have few episodes, spaced years apart, and live normal and productive lives. Others have frequent episodes that result in disability and turmoil. Bipolar disorder can be a serious and sometimes fatal illness; 15 percent of people with it die from suicide. The patient's adherence to treatment may play a large role in determining how they do. Co-morbid substance abuse often predicts a poor outcome. It helped that Josh stopped smoking marijuana and drinking.

For the purposes of our story, we'll assume that Josh did well. He graduated from college and then law school. He married and had four children. He continued to have intermittent episodes of depression, and two of them were severe enough that he had to take a few weeks off work, but he never again needed to be hospitalized.

Chapter 6

Becca:
When Things Go Wrong

SO FAR, we've talked about psychiatry as a discipline that helps people who are suffering from mental disorders, and we've talked about successes. We wish we were able to help every patient we saw, but this is not always how it goes. Recovery is not always a smooth road.

Sometimes, things go wrong. Patients don't get better for many reasons. A person can have an illness that doesn't respond to medications or psychotherapy even when the best treatments are used by the best practitioners and the patient follows instructions exactly. Patients can foil their own care in many ways: missing appointments, not taking medications as prescribed, or abusing drugs and alcohol, to name a few. These are problems that happen even when the psychiatrist does everything right. In this chapter, however, we talk about bad outcomes that happen *because* of the treatment that is rendered.

Treatment can have unexpected outcomes even when the proper care is given. Sometimes the treatment clashes with the patient's expectations. In psychiatry, this can be as simple as a patient's discomfort with a psychiatrist's words—they may leave a patient feeling dismissed, injured, or wronged. Sometimes this occurs because the patient is very sensitive, but other times it happens because the doctor is insensitive, rushed, or even callous. Medications can have side effects and (rarer) adverse reactions, so that even if they are used correctly, symptoms can get worse, or patients may even get ill as a result of their treatment. Psychotherapy that is done poorly can be harmful, and well-meaning psychotherapists can make mistakes because they have inaccurate beliefs about the causes of mental illness. And finally, there are psychiatrists—and we'd like to believe they are few and far between—who violate certain professional standards or boundaries and behave unethically, causing untold injury to their patients.

In chapter 3, we introduced Becca Brandt, the young woman who suffered from borderline personality disorder. Becca was engaging and vivacious, and she became attached to people very easily. Unfortunately, she often felt they let her down, and she was quick to feel slighted and disappointed. Her relationships were often in turmoil, and her moods were labile and tumultuous. Her impulses often got the best of her, and when she was feeling distraught, she was quick to give in to the desire to drink, to have sex with men she barely knew, or even to slice her skin with a razor blade.

We've borrowed Becca to walk through scenarios of psychiatry gone wrong. Some of her difficulties are the result of bad luck—a distressing response to a medication, a miscommunication that leaves her feeling wronged. Other problems are caused by the misguided and unethical behaviors of one of her doctors. Even in the best of circumstances, Becca would not be an easy patient who would find a quick and simple fix, but we have created stories to move her through the worst possible treatment nightmares.

Becca's family was having a difficult time. Her brother Stuart's wife had died in an accident and another brother, Jack, had been diagnosed with cancer. Becca was upset, and she got into arguments with everyone, especially her mother.

"You need to get help, honey," her mother said on the phone one day when Becca was sobbing. It was a conversation they'd had before, and Becca had already seen Dr. Smith and had not found him to be helpful.

"I'd rather die!" Becca yelled at her. She hung up the phone and cut herself on the inside of her upper arm.

Becca eventually consulted Dr. Barbara Stein about her problems, and Dr. Stein recommended that Becca take medication to address her depression, anxiety, and reactive moods. She also recommended psychotherapy to help Becca improve her relationships and find ways to cope with frustration without resorting to self-destructive behaviors. Initially,

Becca went to therapy twice a week, but she refused to take medications. Dr. Stein agreed to see Becca for therapy but said that if this didn't prove to be helpful soon, she hoped Becca would reconsider and try medications, too.

"This is just what I need," Becca said after the third session.

Becca adored Dr. Stein, whom she saw as kind, understanding, smart, and thoughtful. She liked that Dr. Stein was so natural. The psychiatrist didn't wear makeup, always wore comfortable-looking shoes, and kept her hair very short. Becca quickly became attached to her and began calling when she felt upset between sessions. She would contact Dr. Stein when she felt suicidal, or sometimes after she'd cut herself or engaged in a behavior that left her feeling remorseful. Becca did agree to take medication, but she often forgot doses, and she really hated taking it.

Dr. Stein was kind about Becca's frequent calls at first, but it began to feel overwhelming, and Becca's neediness became burdensome.

"I got your message the other evening, and I tried to call you back. It took me a long time to reach you," Dr. Stein said.

"I felt too lousy to talk to anyone, and I turned off the phone," Becca replied.

"I worried about you. You left a message saying you wanted to die, and then you didn't answer the phone. Did you want me to be worried?"

"No. I just didn't want to talk to anyone. And I did call you back later, when I felt better."

What Dr. Stein didn't share with Becca was that situations like this were getting very difficult for her. They happened a lot and felt intrusive. The night in question, Dr. Stein had walked out of her daughter's glee club performance to listen to the phone message, then spent half an hour outside the auditorium trying to return the call, but no one answered. Dr. Stein left the concert and started to drive to her office to get Becca's address so she could send the police to the house, but then Becca left a second message saying she had taken a sleeping pill and was going to bed. She was no longer suicidal. Dr. Stein turned around and got back to the school after the concert was over. She had missed her daughter's solo performance.

After that, Dr. Stein set clearer limits with Becca and asked her not to call between sessions unless she was feeling truly suicidal, in which case it would make sense for Becca to go into the hospital. Becca didn't understand why Dr. Stein was suddenly troubled by her calls. She did, in fact, feel very suicidal at the times she made them, but the feelings passed quickly, and she absolutely wasn't checking herself into a psychiatric unit! Dr. Stein worried that Becca really would kill herself one day, and yet she was exhausted by this patient who seemed to need her so much, so often, and so urgently.

"You don't like me anymore, do you?" Becca asked one day.

Every session was a verbal tug-of-war, and Becca was getting worse, not better. Still, Dr. Stein couldn't tell Becca how frustrated and helpless she felt; such a confession might leave a patient as fragile as Becca feeling even more desperate. Everything about Becca was draining, and Dr. Stein wasn't sure how best to help her.

"You can be a lot of work at times," Dr. Stein answered. At least it felt honest, but the answer upset Becca. Pretty much everything upset Becca, and Dr. Stein was having no luck at getting her to look at how her behavior drew people in then pushed them away.

"Does this feel familiar? Has it happened before that you feel disappointed or hurt by what happens in a relationship?"

"No." Obviously, Becca knew this was a pattern, but she was too angry to admit it.

When Dr. Stein went on vacation, Becca called the doctor who was covering. She'd been drinking, and she told the psychiatrist, "I feel like killing myself now." She'd told this to Dr. Stein many times but then backtracked and assured her that she would not actually kill herself. The covering doctor didn't ask any questions about whether she really intended to commit suicide, and he decided to err on the side of caution by calling the police to have Becca brought to the Emergency Department so she could be evaluated in person. The psychiatrist who saw her in the ED spoke to Dr. Stein's covering psychiatrist and interviewed Becca in detail for forty-five minutes. He determined that she was at low risk for imminent suicide and discharged her home to follow up as an outpatient.

Becca was very angry at Dr. Stein for going away and leaving her to be treated by this other doctor. She felt that he really blew her suicide threat out of proportion. The covering doctor had believed that an emergency evaluation was the prudent thing to do, since he did not know her well, and he'd told her that over the phone. When Dr. Stein returned, Becca was still angry.

"He called the police on me! My neighbors watched them cart me off."

"I'm sorry that happened," Dr. Stein said, "but what was he supposed to do? You called him and said you wanted to kill yourself."

"You're taking his side! You don't understand how wrong this was."

They argued but got nowhere. Dr. Stein explained that Becca's behavior was difficult to deal with. She was often suicidal, presented this as an emergency, wouldn't try certain medications, then wanted her physicians to read her mind and know when the danger was imminent. Becca felt Dr. Stein didn't like her and was dismissive of her distressed feelings over this very upsetting emergency evaluation.

As much as Dr. Stein regretted that she had not been more helpful to Becca, she was relieved when Becca said she was never coming back. She hoped Becca would find a psychiatrist who could help her, but she was also glad for herself that she wouldn't be spending evenings trying to sort out just how dangerous Becca really was.

This is an example of a patient who felt wronged even though the intervention provided was technically correct, although Dr. Stein and the covering psychiatrist could have handled these situations in ways that were more sensitive to Becca's feelings. Sending the police to take a patient to the hospital is never an easy situation. Patients usually feel angry, wronged, and violated, and the distress from this can last a long time. They may direct their anger at the doctor or family member who initiated the police contact and the emergency evaluation. The psychiatrist who was covering for Dr. Stein made a judgment call; he certainly didn't want to make the wrong decision and have Becca die. She felt he should have spent more time talking to her, perhaps offering to see her in his office, and that he should have trusted her not to kill herself. She may have been right that it was unnecessary to send the police. She also thought it was awful that Dr. Stein was no longer willing to talk to her when she was upset after hours, and she was furious that Dr. Stein wouldn't admit that the covering doctor had made a mistake by calling the police. While neither doctor did anything objectively wrong, the patient left treatment feeling angry and injured; she felt no better than she had when she'd first come for help.

Becca decided to see a new psychiatrist, Dr. Amy Wellet, a doctor who specialized in personality disorders. Dr. Wellet reviewed Becca's history and asked Becca if she'd ever been abused.

"My father used to yell at me when I was little. He slapped me a few times." What Becca described was an angry parent, perhaps one who was out of control, but she did not describe abuse of the proportion that leads to severe personality pathology.

"What about sexual abuse?" Dr. Wellet asked.

"Everyone asks me that. I've never been sexually abused."

Dr. Wellet hesitated. "People with your problems have often been traumatized, and they repress these memories. Therapy will help you to remember the abuse and work through it." She sounded quite sure that this was the problem. "The traumas from your past may be causing your personality to split into different segments. You may have different personalities, and this may be why you experience the world in such a wide variety of ways."

Dr. Wellet was certain Becca had repressed memories of sexual abuse, and the doctor was very convincing. It is true that severe personality pathology is often associated with chaotic childhoods and a history of abuse, and for this reason, childhood trauma is considered a risk factor for psychiatric disorders. Not everyone who is traumatized, however, develops pathology, and not everyone with pathology was traumatized. Although Dr. Wellet's theory that Becca was abused and had repressed those memories sounded possible (albeit unprovable), there was no other evidence that Becca had ever been abused. She talked to her parents, her brothers, and extended family members, and they were all certain that she had not been victimized. In the usual scenario, people who have been abused, traumatized, or tortured remember these events clearly, and there is no doubt that they transpired.

"My brothers said we played doctor as kids and I took my shirt off. I was about four then. Could that be the cause of my problems?" Becca asked. Dr. Wellet didn't think so. Becca's symptoms, she said, indicated a severe dissociative disorder and were caused by repeated sexual abuse over time. She pressed Becca to think about this, and Becca thought perhaps there was more to the "playing doctor" scenario than her brothers let on. Her family was appalled when she announced that her oldest brother, Stuart, had sexually molested her, and that as a result, she had developed multiple personalities, each with a different name.

People rarely think of psychotherapy as a treatment that carries risk or that can cause harm, but in fact, any intervention that can heal can also injure. When doctors get informed consent to provide treatment, such as surgery or medications, they talk about these risks with their patients. Just as it's difficult to measure the benefits of psychotherapy, it's also difficult to measure the harm it might cause. This is particularly true for psychotherapy because it isn't the kind of treatment that easily lends itself to scientific measurement of either benefits or harm.

There have been severe instances of therapy gone awry. The most extreme cases are those that are easily recognized as falling outside the realm of treatment—those in which serious boundary violations occur, such as psychiatrists who have sex with their patients or who take financial advantage of their patients. Other examples are therapists who use faddish, trendy, or nontraditional forms of therapy. From the 1980s to the 1990s, there was a movement among some therapists to practice "recovered memory" therapy. This form of therapy was designed to help the supposed victims of child sexual abuse to retrieve memories of the abuse. It was based on the theory that children who have been sexually abused may repress the traumatic memories, and that this causes symptoms and personality dysfunction. Unfortunately, what these therapists neglected to consider was that in certain suggestible patients, it is possible to implant false memories of past events. Patients who fear loss of a therapeutic relationship or who feel pressured to please the therapist may be prone to induced, or suggested, psychiatric syndromes. Induced symptoms can also happen if the patient experiences psychological satisfaction or reward from having the symptoms, for example, by being relieved of unwanted responsibilities or by garnering concern or attention from family members. Becca, in fact, felt encouraged to embrace her newfound memories.

Thus, patients who had never been abused were led to believe that they had been victimized as children, sometimes in bizarre and unimaginable ways. False accusations of sexual abuse led to the breakup of families and even the incarceration of alleged "perpetrators." The recovered memory therapy fad ended only when the patients, after leaving therapy, realized the inaccuracy of their memories. Psychiatric malpractice cases were filed against these therapists and resulted in multimillion-dollar settlements.

The people doing recovered memory therapy, like Dr. Wellet, believed that they were doing psychotherapy properly. Child sexual abuse is a serious problem and can leave lasting psychological effects, but the recovered memory movement is a good example of how well-intentioned therapy can cause harm.

Another, related example of an induced disorder is the syndrome of multiple personality disorder. In the 1990s, an epidemic of cases were being diagnosed even though before that, multiple personality disorder was considered very rare. A review of the medical literature published in 2006 revealed an explosion of scientific interest in the disorder followed by a sharp decline. Hospitals created specialized inpatient units purely for the purpose of treating multiple personality disorder patients, and a specialty journal, *Dissociation*, was created specifically for those involved in the treatment of people with dissociative identity disorder. Some feel it exists as a valid diagnostic entity, while others feel the symptoms can be explained as part of other disorders. Some psychiatrists feel it is not in a patient's best interest to act out different personalities (also called *alters*), and that this behavior may cause uncomfortable responses in those around them.

When Becca announced she had six personalities, all with different names and identities, her family was very skeptical.

"It's like Sybil," her brother Frank said. "Only you don't seem like different people. You seem like one messed-up person! And since you've been seeing that doctor, you've become even more messed up."

Just to clarify, there are certainly many situations in which children were sexually abused or otherwise traumatized and developed psychiatric disorders. Many people have clear memories of being wronged and even tortured, and they are at risk of suffering from disorders such as post-traumatic stress, mood and anxiety problems, and personality vulnerabilities. If someone has memories of these events that have always existed as part of her personal history, psychiatrists don't typically question them. The issue of poor treatment comes up if the memory was "recovered," or implanted, at the suggestion of a therapist when there is no evidence to support a history of abuse.

Some forms of psychotherapy deviate a great deal from mainstream psychiatry, such as past-life regression therapy. These "treatments" may or may not be harmful in and of themselves—we don't know much about them—but they should not be used in place of standard therapies.

How can someone know when therapy is harmful? What should a patient do if she thinks therapy is being done incorrectly, or if she is not sure that what's happening in a session is therapeutic?

It may not be something obvious beyond a general sense that something is happening that makes the patient feel uncomfortable or uneasy. Feeling uneasy doesn't necessarily mean that something improper is happening in treatment. It's possible that the doctor's manner just isn't right for a given patient, as happened between Becca and Dr. Stein. The treatment became uncomfortable, but there was nothing inherently wrong with Dr. Stein's care. Psychotherapy is not always a comfortable process. It's not easy for a patient to hear that he might be at fault when he'd like to blame his micromanaging boss or his lazy wife. The work of psychotherapy can be emotionally trying.

Sometimes a vague feeling of discomfort can evolve into something more extreme. It can be hard to tell when a bad personal fit crosses the line to bad therapy. One sign that things have gone awry is when the therapist becomes locked into one particular theory or explanation of a problem. If a therapist repeatedly insists that the patient's mother is the root of her problems when the patient is certain this is not the case and offers no evidence that it is, this could be a sign that the therapist doesn't have the capacity to re-examine his psychodynamic formulation, or theories of the underlying psychological cause for the patient's problem. Rigid adherence to a psychological theory, despite repeated denials or rejection by the patient, could be a sign that something is going wrong. In the case of the recovered memory therapists, some patients repeatedly denied any history of sexual abuse while their therapists continued to look for clues that it had occurred. Again, this is a difficult issue to define. A patient may suffer from a bizarre delusion, and the therapist may disagree about the validity of the events the patient describes. The psychiatrist may be "rigid" in her formulation that the patient suffers from a psychotic disorder, and in this case, the doctor may be right. If there is doubt, it is important to get information from others.

Another sign that therapy may be going wrong is if a therapist encourages isolation from friends and family in a way that leads the therapist to be a primary or sole source of social support. The goal of therapy is to enhance one's social skills, improve relationships, and broaden social connections. It's not therapeutic to become more locked away and withdrawn.

A typical goal of therapy is to enhance ego strengths, the psychological ability to withstand overwhelming thoughts or feelings. Some types of insight-oriented psychotherapy involve breaking down a patient's defense mechanisms. This type of therapy may cause the patient to regress, and it can be hazardous if done with the wrong person. In this case, the therapy isn't wrong; it just isn't the right treatment for the particular patient.

A therapist who won't consider the use of medication could be practicing inappropriately. In 1984 a malpractice case was filed that was widely discussed in the psychiatric community. *Osheroff v. Chestnut Lodge* involved a patient suffering from clinical depression who was admitted to an inpatient unit and treated only with intensive psychotherapy for many months. His condition worsened, and he was eventually transferred to another facility, where he was treated with medication. Only then did he improve. His lawsuit was settled prior to trial in 1990. This case illustrates the challenge of determining what is or isn't proper therapy—following the Chestnut Lodge settlement, psychiatrists argued among themselves about whether a therapist should be required to consider the use of medication. This case illustrates another unfortunate truth: the standard of practice for psychotherapy is determined more by litigation than by mental health organizations.

Sometimes it may be necessary to change doctors. This is not an easy thing for psychiatric patients to do. It may have been difficult to find a therapist in the first place, or the patient may feel that too much time and energy have been invested in the therapeutic relationship to change. Patients who are symptomatic may be fearful of changing doctors when ill, and they may have to weigh the risk of change versus the risk of staying in a treatment situation that is not working or feels questionable.

Every state has licensing boards and other professional organizations that investigate patient complaints and respond to concerns about questionable therapy. These organizations can require a therapist to seek additional training or supervision, and they can restrict or suspend the license of a therapist who is endangering patients.

Becca thought the idea that she had multiple personalities explained a lot. She started to feel more and more fragile, and her symptoms all became worse, not better. No one else thought she'd been sexually abused during her formative years, and no one seemed to know why she had such problems with her mood and with her behavior. Becca insisted it was because other people pushed her buttons, including her psychiatrists. She decided to stop seeing Dr. Wellet and look elsewhere for help.

Becca went to see a psychiatrist who was strictly a psychopharmacologist and who did not see patients for psychotherapy. This doctor diagnosed Becca with a form of bipolar disorder. Unlike Josh, who was well most of the time and had distinct episodes of depression or mania, Becca had rapid and wide swings in her mood. She was never extremely happy and never had raging energy with a decreased need for sleep, as is typical in mania, but she did have periods when her impulsive behaviors were out of control, and periods when she was depressed and suicidal. One way of thinking about her symptoms was as a primary disorder of her personality, but the psychopharmacologist felt Becca had bipolar disorder type II, with rapid cycling. The type II designation means that patients have episodes of either mood disruption marked by mood elevation or irritability, called *hypomania,* but not to the extreme that they would be called true manic episodes, as in bipolar disorder type I. This doctor thought it might help if Becca's mood were more stable; then her behaviors and reactions might be less extreme. She prescribed a mood stabilizer and an antipsychotic medication. Both medicines helped Becca a great deal, but in a matter of months, she gained twenty pounds and was thirsty all the time. Blood work revealed that Becca had developed diabetes.

Medications are prescribed by doctors to address symptoms, to target abnormal laboratory or radiologic findings, or to prevent the development of disease in at-risk populations, such as aspirin to prevent heart attacks or the ill-fated hormone-replacement therapies that were given to women in the hopes of preventing heart disease and osteoporosis. In short, the point of the medicine is to get rid of something bad or to prevent something worse from happening, and the good thing is that medications often work. In many people, they make the bad symptoms go away, and they allow people to live healthier and longer lives. In patients with psychiatric disorders, medications relieve depression, mania, hallucinations, delusions, and different forms of anxiety. They help people to live fuller lives with less psychic turmoil. The medications Becca took were helpful.

All medications have the potential for side effects, which are usually unwanted symptoms, similar to weeds in a garden. Of course, one person's weed is another person's flower. Skillful doctors will try to take advantage of side effects by matching up a patient's symptoms with common side effects. An example is mirtazapine (Remeron), an antidepressant that causes such side effects as sedation and increased appetite. While this medication is often avoided because of these reactions, in some cases, they are helpful to the treatment, particularly if a patient has lost her appetite and can't sleep.

Mostly, though, side effects are unwelcome. They are uncomfortable for the patient and are often a reason people stop taking medications. Most side effects go away when the medication is stopped, and for some medications, certain side effects are fairly common. Becca had a slight tremor from the mood stabilizer she was taking, but it wasn't bothering her terribly. This side effect would go away if she stopped the medication.

What's interesting about side effects is that few of them happen to everyone. Many people will have sexual difficulties from SSRIs, such as Prozac, but certainly not everyone will. Some people will have a tremor from lithium, as Becca did, and some will get tired on Thorazine. Certain cancer chemotherapies cause nearly everyone who has them to lose their hair, but many side effects seem to be more random. A medication that is associated with a problem such as weight gain won't necessarily cause everyone who takes it to gain weight. Because we cannot accurately predict who will have side effects (just as we can't predict who will have a good therapeutic response), we tell patients about the more frequent side effects with the implicit understanding that other side effects may also occur. The pharmacy distributes a more complete list of potential problems when the medication is dispensed to the patient.

We are now discovering that some side effects may be genetically determined. For example, a certain genetic variant of the GNB3 gene has been weakly associated with antipsychotic-induced weight gain. In the future, we may be able to better predict who will have specific adverse reactions and who will respond to specific medications. For now, we're left to follow reactions in patients and, if they have them, to help them decide if the benefits outweigh the side effects.

There is no guarantee of a free ride: every pill swallowed has the possibility for adverse effects. For the patient who is struggling with a condition that's impeding her life, it may be worth taking the *risk* of a given side effect because that side effect may simply not happen. The problem is what to do when the patient has a good response to the medicine but also has undesirable side effects: unfortunately this scenario leaves the patient and doctor with difficult choices. This is what happened to Becca. She had a good response to the medicines—her mood was better, she was less irritable, and she no longer felt suicidal—but she gained weight and became diabetic.

Side effects are sometimes unpleasant, but many of them are anticipated and reversible. Some medications have rare or really severe effects, which can be debilitating, irreversible, or even fatal. Stevens-Johnson syndrome, liver failure, and agranulocytosis are examples of life-threatening adverse reactions. Stevens-Johnson syndrome is a very rare reaction to a medication, such as lamotrigine (Lamictal), which includes blistering and sloughing of the skin; patients with this syndrome may need treatment in a burn unit. Agranulocytosis is another rare adverse reaction to a medication that causes the bone marrow to shut down and stop making new blood cells. Without white blood cells to mount a response to infection, patients can get sick and die. Agranulocytosis can occur with medicines like clozapine and carbamazepine (Tegretol). Tardive dyskinesia is a movement disorder that develops as an adverse reaction to antipsychotic medications, particularly the older ones. This particular reaction may take years to develop, and it is often irreversible.

Becca's side effect of weight gain and adverse reaction of diabetes gave her a very difficult decision to make. Her psychiatrist encouraged her to substitute another medication that was not as strongly associated with weight gain and diabetes. The new medication was more expensive, and until Becca tried it, she would not know if it would work as well for her.

Severe adverse reactions are sometimes highlighted within black box warnings, labels that the Food and Drug Administration (FDA) requires manufacturers to place on medications when there are severe or life-threatening risks. An example of a black box warning is the one on second-generation antipsychotic medicines that warns about an increased risk of death in elderly patients with dementia who take these medications.

Another black box warning is for the development of suicidal thoughts with antidepressant treatment in people under the age of 25. Becca was not warned about this; however, Josh, the college student who took Zoloft, was told there was a small risk of suicidal thoughts being induced by the medication. Because this adverse reaction has gotten so much attention in the media, we'll discuss it in some detail.

Suicidal thoughts and behaviors are symptoms and signs that are commonly seen in patients with depression. The idea that the medications used to treat depression *cause* suicidal ideas is therefore difficult to assess. To look at this phenomenon, it was necessary to study populations who were depressed but not suicidal. A comprehensive look at the studies revealed that 1 to 2 percent of young people who were not thinking about suicide before treatment started to think about it after beginning an SSRI, usually within the first few days to weeks of treatment.

Prozac has been used by psychiatrists since the late 1980s to treat depression and anxiety disorders. Since we first started using it, there have been questions about what role, if any, it or other SSRIs might have in causing certain patients to become violent. Some families have alleged that the medication precipitated suicidal thoughts and behaviors in their children, and that some suicide deaths were caused by the medication.

Eventually, the FDA began addressing concerns from the general public about the safety of antidepressant medications.

The FDA Advisory Committee on Psychopharmacology convened in December 2006 to listen to the findings of the pharmaceutical agencies, the reports of academic researchers, and the anecdotes of families. One of the coauthors of this book, Dr. Steven Daviss, attended the FDA Advisory Committee meeting and provided testimony. Seventy-five people testified, and the meeting lasted a total of nine and a half hours! Public comments followed, and some of the stories were gut wrenching and impassioned. Because this committee is advisory, the FDA takes what it says into consideration but is not bound by the findings, although the FDA does typically follow the committee's recommendations.

This is what was found: as age goes up, the relative risk of suicidal thoughts *or* suicidal behavior goes down. In other words, younger people are more likely to have suicidal thoughts associated with taking SSRIs. This result supports the decision made in 2004 to add a black box warning stating that these medications are associated with an increase in suicidal thoughts or behavior. (As it turns out, it is just thoughts, not behavior, which we address below.) Note that these events appear to be rare: 12 people out of 3,227 taking medication, and 24 out of 2,397 taking placebo, reported suicidal thoughts or behaviors. For patients over 65, there is clearly a significantly decreased risk of suicidal thoughts or behaviors.

We learned some interesting things by listening to testimony at the FDA Advisory Committee hearings. Sheila Matthews from *AbleChild. org* suggested requiring MedWatch info on all pharmaceutical advertising. MedWatch is the voluntary side-effect-reporting mechanism for the FDA. Few prescribers and fewer consumers use it to report side effects. The FDA should go one step further and make it very easy for consumers to directly report side effects.

Two attorneys brought a number of their clients to testify, and people from the Church of Scientology's Citizen's Commission on Human Rights, despite their reputation, made excellent points about Lilly's unmet promise from fifteen years ago to provide additional data. There were many people who had tragically lost family members who had taken only a few doses of medication. It is indeed hard to understand how a chemical can cause one to conduct such complex, planned behaviors, yet the testimony was compelling, and it did seem as if an idiosyncratic response to a medication might have contributed to these deaths. Joe Glenmullen, author of *Prozac Backlash*, testified as well. He and others stated that the FDA had been tricked by the drug companies, who did not give complete information about all clinical trial results. In fact, the pharmaceutical companies have come under great scrutiny because they publish mostly positive results, not results from studies that show their medications do not work. There is now an online registry at *clinicaltrials. gov* where pharmaceutical companies are expected to post the results of *all* their studies.

The advisory committee deliberated for several hours. All the voting members repeatedly pointed out the importance of balancing any labeling changes—meaning a change in the black box warning already on SSRIs and other antidepressants—with language that emphasized a need to weigh the relative risks of taking the medications against the risk of not taking them, especially since people with untreated depression can be at risk of suicide. When the vote came up about extending the language in the black box to include young adults, two members voted against it, while the other six voted for it with the condition that balancing language be included as well. They told the FDA that they wanted to review the draft language prior to making a final decision.

Then the committee members made several important points:

1. The FDA needs to make the drug companies collect and provide better data.

2. There are inadequate data on the *activation syndrome* induced by antidepressants in some individuals. This activation syndrome consists of physical restlessness, anxiety, and irritability.

3. Collecting pharmacogenetic data might help determine which individuals are at higher risk of developing this and other side effects.

4. The FDA is not collecting adequate data to differentiate between suicidal *thoughts* and suicidal *behaviors* and attempts, so any change in warning language needs to be carefully worded.

5. The committee insisted the FDA add balancing language to reflect not only the increased risk of suicidality in young adults, but also the other side

of the coin—the *increased risk of suicide that is associated with untreated depression.* Additionally, it requested language that refers to the apparent protective effect of these drugs in older adults. This would be the first time the FDA has included information of a positive nature in a black box.

6. The committee was very concerned about the unintended consequences of decreased access to treatment of depression as a result of the black box warning. After the 2004 pediatric black box was added, prescriptions of antidepressants to children decreased, while suicides increased. This trend has already been noted in adults, and the fear is that it will only get worse when the black box warning is extended to young adults.

7. The 25-to-30-year-old group was not chosen scientifically; it just fit the data. There is nothing special that happens when a patient turns 26 or 31 to alter risk. Because of this, the committee considered using the nonspecific term "young adults," but this idea wasn't very popular.

8. Some of the possible explanations discussed for the biphasic nature of the data—that is, the higher risk when younger and lower risk when older—included induction of mania; late maturation of frontal lobes of the brain, decreasing impulsivity as people get older; and greater tolerance of uncomfortable emotions that may come with age. The committee agreed that more data would be helpful.

9. The committee also felt it was very important to emphasize the need for close follow-up when treating people of *any* age with depression. There was concern that it could sound like older people don't need to be followed as closely due to this protective effect.

10. Finally, the FDA acknowledged concern about telling doctors how to practice medicine. However, it was pointed out that when the stakes have been high enough, the FDA has dictated the frequency of monitoring lab tests. Telling prescribers that depressed patients who are starting antidepressants should be followed at least weekly in the beginning should be no different.

Josh did not become suicidal as a result of taking Zoloft. Becca was not so lucky in avoiding adverse reactions. Her diabetes developed after starting Zyprexa, also called olanzapine. Her blood sugar quadrupled, and she was treated in an emergency room with intravenous fluids and insulin, then started on a medication for diabetes. She was left to decide, along with her family and doctor, whether she wanted to continue taking the medication that had been so helpful or to stop it in the hopes that the diabetes would resolve and another medication would be just as helpful without this reaction.

"I knew this was a risk," Becca said. "I just thought it was a small risk, and I didn't think it would happen to me."

Sometimes patients feel angry when they experience a side effect or an adverse reaction they were not warned about. The list of possible side effects can be very long, and some people experience problems that have not been reported. It's the usual standard to warn patients about the more common side effects and about any black box warnings that have been issued by the FDA. Some doctors choose to be quite inclusive while others give little information about side effects and expect patients to review the package insert provided by the pharmacy. Usually, doctors do warn patients that a mood stabilizer, such as the lithium that Becca was taking, can cause harm to the thyroid and kidneys, and that the function of these organs has to be monitored regularly with blood tests as long as the patient remains on the medication. The second-generation antipsychotics have been implicated in various metabolic problems, including weight gain, diabetes, and elevated cholesterol levels, and these conditions also need to be monitored.

Becca's doctor made her aware of these risks. She and Becca decided to stop the antipsychotic agent and see how Becca did on the mood stabilizer alone. Becca could take a second medication, the more expensive antipsychotic agent, if she felt she needed it during difficult periods. Becca did fine on this regimen, but she still had difficulties with her relationships and still felt she was not able to accomplish as much as she wanted. Her psychopharmacologist suggested she resume psychotherapy.

Dr. Janice Williamson was a charming lady, and Becca found her office interesting. She displayed artwork from all over the world, and she enjoyed telling Becca about her trips. Becca had traveled with her family to many of the same places, so they had this in common. Sometimes, the sessions would run over by fifteen or twenty minutes, and they would talk about any number of things. Becca knew that Dr. Williamson was going through a divorce and was also taking medication for depression. Becca liked Dr. Williamson's warmth and openness, and she liked that she wasn't withholding like Dr. Stein, pushy like Dr. Wellet, or "just medicines and symptoms" like the psychopharmacologist. It felt like a good match to Becca.

Things changed quickly. One day Dr. Williamson looked out of sorts, and Becca asked if she was okay.

"Pulled my back," the doctor said.

"You look uncomfortable. I just stopped at the drugstore to pick up my brother's prescriptions, and he takes something for pain. I'm sure he'd be fine if I gave you a few." Becca's brother, Jack, was still undergoing treatment for lymphoma, and the whole family was helping with his care. Dr. Williamson reluctantly took a couple of the pain pills.

The following week, Becca asked Dr. Williamson about her back pain. It was still troubling her, but those pills had helped.

"You know, Janice," Becca said, "You really should see a doctor about this and get some medication."

"I am a doctor!" Janice Williamson said.

"Well, why don't you write yourself a prescription?" Becca asked.

"It's not legal to write for narcotics for yourself," Dr. Williamson replied.

"Well, I'm your patient. You could write a prescription for me, and I could give the pills to you."

This relationship was set on a path for disaster. Becca became her psychiatrist's vehicle for a narcotic habit, and she soon felt angry and used. She made demands of Dr. Williamson, who was now afraid that if she didn't provide whatever Becca wanted, Becca would report her to the medical licensing board or sue her. Becca asked for a prescription for Xanax, and she became angry when Dr. Williamson wanted to end the sessions on time or didn't want to meet her for coffee between sessions.

"My brother is really sick, and you only care about me when I'm getting you Percocet!" Becca howled. She'd been doing so well, but she stopped seeing the psychopharmacologist, stopped taking the medications, and was more fragile than she'd ever been. Dr. Williamson had stopped being part of the solution and became part of the problem.

All relationships have boundaries for what is and is not acceptable in terms of behavior. In psychotherapy, these boundaries are particularly important for several reasons. For one thing, the rules help define the relationship as something that is different from a friendship or a mentoring relationship. For another, they help keep the focus on the patient and the work of solving his problems or treating his illness. And finally, they help keep the setting safe emotionally and physically. Because psychotherapy is such an intimate and personal endeavor, both the patient and the therapist can be susceptible to feelings and behaviors that may exploit a patient's vulnerability. Boundaries keep this from happening.

Some common therapeutic boundaries include the following:

- The sessions take place in the psychiatrist's office. (It may be a home office.)
- The length of the session is decided in advance, and the patient stays only for the length of the session.
- The doctor is paid for the treatment.
- Physical contact is limited to a handshake and the necessary maneuvers related to medical treatment, for example, the contact required to take a pulse or blood pressure.
- Medication is prescribed by the psychiatrist for specific reasons, and addictive medicines are tightly controlled by the prescriber.
- Therapists and patients don't typically exchange gifts, at least not of any significant monetary value.
- Psychiatrists and their patients do not get together for social events. This doesn't mean they can't speak at a party, but they don't plan meetings for social purposes.
- The amount of personal information the psychotherapist is expected to disclose is limited, although an exact boundary for therapist self-disclosure is not defined by any consensus. While some psychiatrists may choose to tell patients where they went on vacation or whether they have children, it would never be acceptable for a psychiatrist to discuss details of his sexual life with a patient.
- Some psychotherapists, particularly psychiatrists, may prefer to address patients by their last names as a statement of the professional nature of the relationship.

- In psychotherapy, everyone remains dressed, and violence on the part of either party is never acceptable. Typically, the existence of a psychotherapeutic relationship excludes the possibility of an intimate, outside-the-office friendship, and psychiatrists are not permitted to have sexual relationships with patients, even after the termination of the therapeutic relationship.

These boundaries are general guidelines, and there are certainly circumstances when they need to be approached with thoughtful consideration, or even broken. If the psychiatrist extends the length of the session because the patient needs to be hospitalized, this would not be a boundary violation. Sometimes a patient can't afford treatment, and a psychiatrist chooses to decrease or waive the fee. As long as other boundaries are in place, this would not be considered anything other than generous. There are moments when holding to designated boundaries may be awkward or even harmful, and the psychiatrist is left to his best judgment.

In the movies, psychiatrists often violate professional boundaries in outrageous and provocative ways. It is not unheard of for psychiatrists and patients to have romantic relationships, however, and for these relationships to be the subject of professional and ethical investigations. And boundaries violations are not issues only for psychiatrists. They can occur in any type of relationship where there is an imbalance of power. In any doctor-patient, teacher-student, employer-employee, clergy-congregant dyad, there is the potential for abuse of power. Sometimes it seems like such stories are in the newspaper every day.

Therapeutic boundaries are not hard and fast, and they are not generally designated by law; they can be a bit fluid and open to interpretation. There is nothing specifically illegal about meeting a patient outside the office, and one could imagine a scenario where this would be fine—for example, in an outreach, team-based approach for patients who are unable to keep appointments. There may be other circumstances in which a psychiatrist's insistence on maintaining boundaries could be construed as cold or rejecting, for example, refusing to accept a homemade gift or thrusting a patient away as she offers an unexpected, and perhaps unwelcome, hug. These are difficult situations for the psychiatrist, and there may not be an absolute "right" thing to do.

There may well be nothing inherently wrong with meeting a patient for a social interaction, and the event may proceed as a fond and benign memory for both parties. The risk, however, is that once one artificial boundary is violated, it becomes easier for the psychotherapist to lose sight of what is and isn't acceptable in a professional therapeutic relationship and to pull the relationship even further from the usual standards. This situation is referred to as a slippery slope, where one transgression leads to another and a poor outcome eventually becomes inevitable, such as the case with Becca procuring narcotics for her doctor. Boundary violations where the therapist uses her power for personal fulfillment are always unacceptable. Dr. Williamson and Becca certainly violated a number of the usual boundaries, and the relationship was not about helping Becca.

Suppose a circumstance arose in which the therapist was justified in transgressing certain boundaries, and no difficulties arose. But suppose that the patient later asserted that she was harmed by the psychiatrist's real, imagined, or fabricated indiscretion. Then the credibility of both the accuser and the accused may be called into question. A psychiatrist who openly violated standard boundaries, even if seemingly inconsequential, is more likely to be considered guilty. Thus, a patient who accuses a therapist of sexual misconduct might be more readily believed if the therapist has a history of extending sessions, not collecting fees, meeting the patient outside the office socially, or exchanging expensive gifts.

The intimacy of the therapeutic setting, one in which the therapist and patient are alone together discussing the patient's most personal feelings, can lead to romantic feelings and attachments. The patient, in this setting, may be vulnerable to such feelings. Therapists who are themselves troubled or having difficulties in their personal lives may also find themselves vulnerable to these emotions. For many therapeutic boundaries, it is possible to think of a scenario where transgression is acceptable. There are, however, no situations in which it is ever acceptable for a psychiatrist to have sexual contact with a patient, and these are the instances that cause patients irreparable harm. Psychiatrists who have romantic or sexual relationships with patients are subject to review and censure by professional and licensing organizations, civil lawsuits, and public scrutiny and embarrassment.

Although Becca and Dr. Williamson did not have a romantic relationship, Becca's doctor clearly exploited her. When Becca mentioned what she was doing with the pain medication to her brother Frank, the police officer who was studying to be a social worker, he reported Dr. Williamson to the physician licensing board. She lost her medical license and was the subject of a criminal investigation.

Becca had one bad treatment story after another. Please remember that neither she nor her doctors are real, and that we created a character with many extremes to illustrate the point that things don't always go well. It's a chapter we write with some hesitation—there are already plenty of stories of psychiatry gone wrong out there, and much of it is built up by the media, yet psychiatrists and their patients are rarely portrayed in a positive light. But this book wouldn't be a fair or accurate portrayal of psychiatry if we didn't discuss the bad as well as the good. Patients have illnesses that can be difficult to treat. Our medications don't always work, and sometimes they hurt. Therapy is an intimate process, and even when it's done right, people can be very sensitive to words that are said; meanings can be perceived or misperceived; and interpersonal chemistry can be crucial. Therapy done wrong can be harmful, and there are psychiatrists whose personal issues prevent them from practicing in a safe and healing style.

Chapter 7

Eddie:
A Child at Risk

BY THE TIME Eddie Banks was 7 years old, his mother, Susan, was suffering from advanced AIDS. Susan was a former drug addict who had been estranged from her own family for many years. When Eddie was 18 months old, he was taken from her and placed in foster care, while Susan went to rehab and got clean. After her release, Susan managed to get her life together to regain custody of her son, and once she was clean and employed, Susan reconnected with her own mother, Carolyn. Carolyn was thrilled to meet her only grandson, and things went well for a couple of years, but then Susan was diagnosed with AIDS, and her health declined rapidly. She was in and out of the hospital, and she and Eddie had to move in with Carolyn. Finally, it became clear that Susan was too ill to go home from the hospital and that she would need hospice care.

Susan tried to get out of bed to leave. "I have to get the car," she told the nurse who found her on the floor after she fell. "I've got to pick Eddie up at school!"

Susan hadn't owned a car in nearly two years, and she couldn't walk without assistance, so she certainly couldn't drive. She wanted to be released, and she was refusing treatment.

"My boy needs me. He hasn't got anyone else," Susan said later, after she was settled back in bed. She spit out the medication the nurse gave her. "Enough!" Susan said.

"He'll come home with me, like he always does," said Carolyn. Carolyn reached over the rail of the hospital bed and took Susan's hand. A retired school administrator, Carolyn was a thin and immaculately dressed woman. She'd spent years worrying about Susan, and it had taken a toll on her. Carolyn appreciated how hard Susan's recovery had been, how much she loved Eddie, and how unfair it was that Susan had worked so hard only to lose everything. And Carolyn knew that Eddie needed his grandmother. She was determined to stay in his life, particularly since Lou, Eddie's father, was incarcerated for drug distribution.

Sometimes people become too ill to make decisions about their own health care, or at least to make the decisions they would make when well. When that happens, medical decisions must be made by someone acting on behalf of the patient. Susan had already talked to her mother about her medical care, and she trusted Carolyn to make good choices about recommended medications and procedures. In legal terminology, Carolyn was Susan's *health care proxy*, the person legally designated to make medical decisions for her.

The use of a health care proxy is contingent upon decision-making incompetence. This means that a physician has evaluated the patient and found her to be mentally unable to make choices about medical treatment. For example, if a medical patient is severely demented, or in a coma, and needs to have a surgical procedure, the patient's surgeon would ask a consultation-liaison psychiatrist to see the patient to assess her competence. In many jurisdictions, a finding of incompetence must be based on the assessments of two physicians. Regardless, to find someone incompetent, the physicians must certify that the patient is unable to understand the risks, benefits, and alternatives to the proposed treatment or is unable to communicate the treatment decision.

Once the patient is certified as medically incompetent, the treating physician is allowed to seek a treatment decision from the health care proxy. State law may determine who is designated as the proxy, but it's usually a spouse or other family member. Someone other than a family member could be appointed if the family member is unable or unwilling to act as proxy or if there is evidence that the member is not acting in the patient's best interests. In that case, the hospital would have to go to court to seek appointment of a legal guardian for the patient.

This is a complicated process. Unfortunately, most people don't plan for this situation unless they are making a will or caring for elderly relatives. Attorneys who specialize in estate planning or elder law can give advice about setting up a power of attorney, a legal document, signed in front of witnesses and notarized, that names a patient's health care decision maker. Another type of legal health care document, called an *advance directive*, lists instructions from the patient to the doctor about how she would want her health care decisions made under certain future circumstances, for example, whether to provide fluids and nutrition or to continue mechanical ventilation or other extraordinary measures.

Advance directives are now also being used for decisions about psychiatric treatment. Because it's an emerging area of law, state laws may vary regarding the validity of these directives. A psychiatric advance directive is written and signed by the patient when the patient is well and competent to make decisions, but it is only used when the patient is ill and unable to make decisions. In general, a psychiatric advance directive contains the following information: a statement regarding whom the patient would like to have as proxy, the signature of that person agreeing to act as proxy, the patient's wishes regarding certain types of treatment (hospitalization, use of medications or electroconvulsive therapy, and use of seclusion and restraint), and the conditions under which the patient would want the advance directive terminated. More information about advance directives, including sample forms, can be obtained from the National Resource Center on Psychiatric Advance Directives.

Carolyn was already designated as Susan's health care proxy, and there were documented advance directives in Susan's medical chart. She didn't want any invasive procedures or life-sustaining measures. She had already been through enough. When Susan refused treatment, no one forced the issue, and she was much too weak to even try to get to the long-gone car or to have any influence over Eddie's day-to-day actions. What wasn't yet clear was what would happen to Eddie after she died. She didn't want to think about it, and she avoided talking to Carolyn or to Eddie about the future. That was still the state of affairs when, several weeks later, Susan died at the hospice.

Unfortunately, many families have challenging and difficult social situations in this country, and adult problems like poverty, substance abuse, mental illness, and criminal activity all have an effect on children. These problems bring children into contact with the court system through no fault of their own. Some children are abandoned or neglected, or have parents who are unable to care for them for various reasons. The state grants the court power to intervene in these cases. The court, acting under *parens patriae* (in the place of the parent) powers, may take the child under its legal custody to remove him from the home, or to coerce the parents into treatment. By the turn of the twentieth century, many states charged child welfare agencies with the management of neglected and abused children. The judicial system created juvenile courts to address the needs of these children and their families. The idea behind this was that the children were at risk for developing future criminal behavior and that early intervention could prevent this.

Susan had not designated a guardian for Eddie. His father was in prison, and there was no contact with Lou's family. The only reasonable guardian was Carolyn, and she was devoted to Eddie. He remained with her.

No one had an easy time of it. Carolyn's health was poor, and Eddie was a lot of work. He missed his mother terribly, and he struggled in school. By the time he was nine, he was skipping school, and before he was twelve, he was hanging out on the streets with older, streetwise teenagers, defying all authority and living by his own rules. Carolyn tried to talk to him—indeed, thinking of Susan's past difficulties, she begged and pleaded with Eddie—but nothing she said or did changed his behavior. He was out of control, and she took him to a children's mental health center for counseling.

Dr. Marilyn Peabody was soft-spoken and gentle. She met with Carolyn first and learned about Eddie's birth, developmental years, medical history, and recent problems. Then she met with Eddie and was immediately struck by his constant curiosity and activity. Instead of sitting next to his grandmother on a chair, he made a beeline for the small bookcase next to Dr. Peabody's desk and methodically began pulling the books off the shelves one by one. When Carolyn tried to intervene, he glared at her, shrugged, picked up a small rubber ball and began bouncing it off the wall. Helplessly, Carolyn turned to Dr. Peabody. "See? This is the reaction I get. He doesn't listen. He shrugs. Sometimes he throws things or curses at me. I give him everything he needs, but this is what happens. I'm afraid of the trouble he'll get into if he keeps spending time with those kids on the corner. Can you help us?"

Dr. Peabody was very familiar with the trouble found on the streets of a large urban city. She asked more questions to see how far his behavior problems went.

"Does he listen to teachers? How does Eddie get along with other children? Does he act on impulse, blurt out answers, or have trouble waiting his turn? Does Eddie have a short fuse? Has he used any street drugs? Has he ever run away from home? Does Eddie get into fights?"

Dr. Peabody asked these questions because she knew that some at-risk children are already involved in behaviors that are indicators of future trouble, such as running away from home or staying out past curfew. Like Eddie, they might be generally disobedient and talk back to or swear at their parents and teachers. If the behaviors are severe, persistent, and dangerous enough, or if there is reason to believe there is parental neglect or abuse, these children can be removed from the home and placed in foster care. Courts then put together a remediation plan: a treatment or rehabilitation plan for the family, with the goal of family reunification. The remediation plan may mandate counseling for the parents and child, drug treatment, rehabilitation, psychiatric treatment, or parenting classes. If the parents make good faith efforts to follow the plan, they retain parental rights. If they fail to follow the plan, or if intervention doesn't work after repeated efforts, the child may be permanently removed from the home. Parental rights can be terminated, meaning that the parents have no legal authority to make decisions for the child or even have contact with him, but this rarely happens except in cases of severe abuse or outright abandonment, when the child is placed for adoption. Eddie had been the victim of neglect at a very early age, but there was no reason to believe that his grandmother was in any way abusive or neglectful. In this setting, the issue was simply one of getting him help, and there was no need for the legal system to be involved.

Carolyn did her best to answer the doctor's questions, but to get the full picture, Dr. Peabody had to talk to his teacher. After considering all this information, Dr. Peabody was able to make a diagnosis of attention deficit hyperactivity disorder. She talked to Carolyn about a treatment plan, including family therapy with a social worker in the clinic, a behavior plan for Eddie, and the option of treatment with medication.

"Do I have to agree to the medication in order for him to get it?" Carolyn asked.

"Yes," said Dr. Peabody. "If he were older, say, age 16, he would be able to agree to treatment on his own, but he's too young for that now."

The age of consent for medical or mental health care is an aspect of juvenile law that can vary from state to state. The idea that juveniles might have a right to consent to treatment independent of parental consent is a relatively new idea, as is the idea of juvenile rights in general. Under old English common law, a man's house, farm, crops, cattle, wife, and children were considered "chattel," or property. Marriages were arranged as business deals, a means of acquiring property or forming political alliances with influential officials. Women and children were the bargaining chips of these alliances. Children cemented marital agreements over the long term by guaranteeing a line of ownership for land holdings. They were also the unpaid labor of colonial America. They were sent away to serve uncompensated apprenticeships or hired to work long hours in factories during the Industrial Revolution. The children of poor families were sent to workhouses with their parents and siblings to work off family debts.

This changed as a result of the social reform movement in the mid to late nineteenth century. Reformers like Dorothea Dix lobbied Congress to set aside land for state psychiatric hospitals to care for the mentally ill. Other reformers founded schools to educate emancipated slaves, and women banded together to start the women's suffrage movement. For the first time, children were considered to have individual rights and interests separate from their parents. Over the course of the twentieth century, laws were developed to address children's access to education; parental custody; abuse, abandonment, or neglect; and due process protections in criminal proceedings and laws regulating the mental health treatment of juveniles. Family law became a legal specialty.

Parents are responsible for making decisions regarding the rearing, discipline, and health care of their children, but even parents have state-imposed limits on what they're allowed to do. For example, they can choose a specific school for a child to attend, but they cannot choose to deny education. They can choose whether or not their child can have elective surgery but not to withhold life-saving procedures. They can punish a child but not through physical abuse or starvation. State laws set limits on parental authority for the protection of the child.

Children have medical privacy rights and may also be able to give independent consent for treatment depending on their age. The age of consent for treatment varies between states but is generally between 13 and 16 years. Once the age of consent is reached, the child may independently receive prenatal care or birth control as well as treatment for sexually transmitted diseases or mental health or substance abuse issues. Laws regarding medical confidentiality and medical consent still apply when the child is not under the legal control of a parent. A child under the guardianship of a child welfare agency retains his right to privacy. This means that the guardian or agency must give consent for access to the child's treatment records.

Having the right to give medical consent does not mean the child has unlimited treatment rights. Parental notification laws may limit independent consent for abortion in some states. And independent consent also does not exempt the clinician from mandatory reporting laws for child abuse—so a therapist may still be required to report abuse even if the child wants it to remain confidential.

Juveniles have other age-dependent rights, such as the right to be employed or to have a driver's license. The required age of consent for these activities varies quite a bit between states. Even within the same state, the age of consent for legal drinking may be different from the age of consent to have a driver's license or to have sex. And all these ages may be different from the age of majority, the age at which a juvenile legally becomes an adult. In most states now the age of majority is 18. A child can also legally become an adult if he is emancipated—officially declared independent from his parents. To do this, the juvenile must prove that he has lived away from his parents for a significant amount of time and that he has not relied on them for material support. Parents must be given notice that the child is seeking emancipation, and they have a right to challenge this at a hearing.

Carolyn agreed to Dr. Peabody's treatment plan and did her best to get Eddie to go along with it as well. Unfortunately, she had trouble getting him to family therapy sessions. Some days he wouldn't come home from school in time for the appointments, and other days he simply refused to go. He also refused to take the medication that Dr. Peabody prescribed, and he generally came and went from home as he pleased. The situation came to a head when Carolyn got a call from the local police precinct.

"What has he done now?" she asked, exasperated. The police officer on the other end of the line obviously had a great deal of experience talking to overwhelmed parents. Patiently, he explained that Eddie and two of his teenage friends were suspected of burglarizing a local business. The officer needed Carolyn to come and take Eddie home until a hearing could be held.

"Is he under arrest? What is he charged with?" she asked.

"Well, he's a juvenile, so we can't charge him with anything, ma'am, but he is going to have to go to juvenile court and appear in front of a judge because of what happened. You might want to talk to a lawyer."

Carolyn was confused about why she would need a lawyer if Eddie wasn't charged with a crime. What Carolyn didn't know was that according to the laws of most states, children under a certain age are thought to be too young to form the *intent*, or mental state, required to commit a crime, so they cannot be brought before a criminal court for their behavior. By legal tradition, that cut-off age is 7 years; however, it may be defined differently by state statute. Children older than age 14 can be charged with crimes according to most state laws. In between the ages of seven and fourteen, juveniles can be brought before a court and held responsible for their behavior. This is done through the juvenile justice system rather than the adult criminal justice system.

A juvenile, such as Eddie, accused of a criminal act goes before a juvenile court through delinquency proceedings rather than through a criminal prosecution. First, a delinquency petition is filed, which documents the facts of the alleged offense. The child has many of the same due process rights available to adult criminals, including the right to counsel and to notice about the hearing, the right to call and cross-examine witnesses, and the right to examine the evidence against him. If the juvenile judge decides that the youngster committed the offense, he is considered an adjudicated delinquent rather than a convicted criminal. Juveniles can't be found "guilty" in the juvenile justice system since they are thought to be incapable of forming the mental intent to commit a crime.

Once there is a finding of delinquency, the court holds another hearing, called a disposition hearing, to figure out what to do with the child. Generally, the disposition plans are very similar to what happens when children are placed in foster care in that a treatment plan is developed with the goal of family reunification. Rarely, the child is placed in a specialized juvenile rehabilitation or treatment facility. Institutionalization is not the first choice for a number of reasons. Juveniles are more likely to reform if they maintain family contact and support, especially if the family unit is responsible and stable. Also, inpatient rehabilitation programs are hard to come by, so they are reserved for juveniles who represent a high risk of danger to public safety. If the juvenile is repeatedly delinquent, the juvenile justice system has the option of passing responsibility from juvenile court to adult criminal court. This process, also known as a juvenile waiver, is an admission that the juvenile can no longer be rehabilitated through the juvenile system.

Certain crimes are defined by law as automatic adult offenses. In other words, these crimes are so serious that a juvenile over the age of 14 will automatically be charged in the adult criminal justice system. These offenses include crimes like murder, rape, arson, or felony drug distribution. The juvenile's attorney has the option of asking that jurisdiction be moved back to juvenile court in a process known as transfer of jurisdiction.

Carolyn hired an attorney to help her negotiate Eddie's case. At the delinquency hearing, the judge listened to the juvenile state's attorney present the case, then Eddie's lawyer spoke to the judge. The judge listened carefully and eventually decided there was enough evidence to support a finding of delinquency. He released Eddie to the care of his grandmother and placed him on one year of juvenile probation. As part of the probation agreement, Eddie was required to get counseling, take any recommended psychiatric medication, attend school, and keep the curfew his grandmother had set up. A probation agent was appointed through the juvenile services agency to monitor Eddie's progress and to stay in touch with Carolyn.

"This is serious, Eddie. You have to do what the judge says," Carolyn told him.

Forensic psychiatrists are involved in many aspects of juvenile rehabilitation in both the juvenile and the adult justice systems. They help set up rehabilitation plans for delinquent children and family reunification plans for children in foster care. They assess juvenile competency, or mental fitness, to participate in delinquency proceedings. They also provide input to the court about which justice system is most appropriate for the juvenile. They sometimes provide the psychiatric care for institutionalized delinquents. In the story we've just told, Eddie had no contact with a forensic psychiatrist. Although everyone was worried about him, he'd committed a nonviolent crime with friends; it was his first offense; and there was no need for foster care or detention.

Eddie's situation became more complicated when his father, Lou, was released from prison on parole. Shortly after his release, Lou went to Carolyn's home and demanded that Eddie come with him, to stay in the apartment that he and his new girlfriend shared. Carolyn was horrified.

"You can't take him just like that!" she said. "He hasn't seen you in years, and he barely remembers you! If you want to come in and visit, that's fine, but we have to think about what's best for Eddie."

Lou relented and came in to see his son for the first time in years. Eddie was reluctant to visit and resisted any questions about school, friends, or activities. Lou tried to talk to him about changing homes.

"You see, I'm your father. You need a man in your life. Your grandma is a good lady, but she can't take care of you like I can."

At that point Eddie ran to his room, and Carolyn told Lou the visit was over.

"He'll be coming with me," Lou said. "You just wait. It's gonna happen."

Three weeks later, Carolyn received a summons for a custody hearing.

Custody issues usually come up in the setting of divorce. It's an unfortunate reality that thousands of divorces take place every month. Fortunately, most are settled by mutual agreement, and court involvement is a formality to finalize the divorce decree. Even when children are involved, most custody and visitation agreements get worked out between the parties as part of the separation. Amicable settlements are also reached through informal mediation in some cases. In other words, the couple meets with someone other than a judge or lawyer to negotiate the terms of the divorce, including custody and visitation arrangements. However, extended conflict can occur over child custody when one parent alleges domestic violence or child abuse, or when a parent suffers from mental illness or substance abuse. When this happens, the court may order a psychiatric evaluation to determine which custody arrangement is in the best interest of the child. In Eddie's case, the issue of custody came up when his father was released from prison and decided he wanted to resume his role as parent.

Custody evaluations are difficult cases for a forensic evaluator to do because these cases tend to be complex and because the welfare of a child is at stake. A custody evaluation involves interviews with many people—with the parents and each child, and sometimes with friends and relatives or other people who have information relevant to the parties' parenting capacity. A custody evaluation may also involve psychological tests of each involved party. The evaluator considers each child individually and looks at factors such as the child's developmental, psychological, and medical issues, and educational needs. The evaluator considers the child's personality and temperament, hobbies or other interests, and needs for structure and supervision. If the child has exhibited conduct problems, the evaluator also considers the child's response to discipline. Depending on the child's age, he may be asked directly which parent he wants to live with. The custody laws of some states require courts to consider the child's preference.

The custody evaluator will do an extensive psychiatric interview with each litigant. In addition to all the usual questions asked during a psychiatric evaluation, the custody evaluator will ask many questions about the parent's own developmental history and parenting experience. The evaluator will pay particular attention to aspects of the parent's history that relate to substance abuse and criminal involvements as well as physical or psychiatric conditions that may affect parenting capacity. Finally, the evaluator will assess the parent's understanding of the child's needs.

These are some of the questions the evaluator asks himself to form an opinion about custody:

- Does this parent understand where the child is developmentally? Does he use discipline appropriate for that developmental level?
- Does this parent have the ability to put the child's needs above his own interests?
- Is he capable of providing for the financial and medical needs of the child?
- Has he considered the child's relationship with the noncustodial parent, and is he willing to support that relationship?
- Has this parent considered where the child will go to school?
- Has this parent made arrangements for the child's living space, travel to school, and travel to visitation?

The results of any psychological tests will also be considered; however, psychological testing alone does not predict or correlate with parental fitness. The purpose of psychological testing in custody evaluations is mainly to identify any gross pathology that may affect parenting ability.

Once all this information is gathered and considered, the evaluator makes a recommendation about custody based on the legal standard of that particular jurisdiction. In the nineteenth century, courts followed the paternal preference standard, which automatically granted custody to the father. This was consistent with the idea that children, like other marital property, belonged to the husband. Any woman who divorced her husband automatically lost access to her children. Eventually this changed to a maternal preference standard, in which just the opposite occurred, and fathers lost custody automatically. Most recently, court cases established the idea of the *psychological parent*, an acknowledgment that a child could be emotionally bonded to an adult who was not a biological parent. The current and most recent standard for determining child custody is known as the *best interests of the child* standard. Using this standard, child custody is based not on any predetermined parental preference but on the best fit between the custodial parent and the child. This is the prevailing standard for most states now. Occasionally a guardian *ad litem*—an attorney chosen by the court—is appointed to represent the child's interests.

The court must make decisions regarding both the legal and the physical custody of the child, and these are generally awarded to the same person. There are many possible arrangements for custody, however. The most common form of custody now is joint, in which both parents share legal custody, and the living situation of the child is shared between households. Sole or full custody is when a single parent is awarded all rights to make legal decisions for the child, and the noncustodial parent is allowed visitation. Third-party custody is a relatively new idea, when custody is awarded to someone other than a biological parent—for example, to grandparents, gay partners, or another interested party. Split custody has sometimes been used interchangeably with joint custody, but it actually refers to an arrangement in which siblings are separated from one another, and custody is awarded to different parents. Finally, temporary custody may be granted to a parent if the other parent is briefly incapacitated or unavailable, such as by illness or incarceration.

As society changes and new social settings arise, custody law must evolve to account for them. In vitro fertilization caused courts to consider which parent has the right to claim custody or use of frozen embryos. The use of surrogate mothers necessitated legal arrangements to clarify parental rights over the child. No doubt we will see other developments in family law as family life reconfigures and reproductive technology evolves.

To finish up Eddie's story for this chapter, we're going to assume that Eddie and his family lived in a state that, by law, didn't recognize the custodial rights of grandparents. After a prolonged hearing with much testimony, including a court-ordered custody evaluation with testimony by the forensic psychiatrist, the family court judge decided that legal and physical custody of Eddie would return to Lou. As one might expect, this increased the instability in Eddie's life. How Eddie's life continues is the subject of chapter 8.

Chapter 8

Eddie:
The Prison Patient

EDDIE HAD A traumatic and challenging childhood. His early years were marked by instability, bad influences, and poor choices. Before he turned 12, Eddie came into contact with the court system through a juvenile burglary. As a result of this delinquency hearing, he was required to attend outpatient counseling and to pay restitution for the damage he had caused to the business he burglarized.

We used Eddie's case to describe some of the legal issues that involve the participation of forensic psychiatrists. Juveniles are usually involved in issues that are civil matters, such as decisions about child custody and visitation or child neglect proceedings. Juvenile delinquency hearings are also technically civil in nature because the purpose of the process is to provide treatment and rehabilitation to juvenile offenders rather than punishment. However, forensic psychiatrists also work with people who become involved in criminal legal issues. Criminal law pertains only to people who are legally adults. Although it would be nice to give Eddie's story a happy ending, we're going to walk him through more trouble to illustrate how forensic psychiatrists become involved in the criminal arena.

Unfortunately, Eddie's father, Lou, was no believer in mental health services. He didn't like the idea of having his child "drugged up" on psychiatric medications, and because he was only occasionally employed, he couldn't afford to keep Eddie in counseling. By the time Eddie was 18, he was over six feet tall and weighed 180 pounds. Eddie and Lou fought frequently, both verbally and physically. One night Eddie took off for good when Lou was sleeping. On his way out the door, he took Lou's cocaine and heroin, then broke into an abandoned building to share the drugs with his friend Bernie. Police cruising the area saw the building's front door broken off its hinges and found Bernie and Eddie nodding off in an upstairs bedroom. They were both charged with breaking and entering and drug possession, misdemeanor crimes.

When Eddie went to court, he admitted he had a drug problem. "I need help," he said to the judge. "I can do probation, and I'll even go back to the clinic I was in before. I quit taking my medication and got depressed. At the clinic they told me I was self-medicating." Eddie's public defender knew about his drug problem and his psychiatric history. He knew that the best outcome for his client would be to get Eddie involved in a specialty court designed for offenders like him, and he told Eddie his plan to ask the judge to transfer the case to mental health court.

Specialty courts were created because judges recognized that certain types of offenders had conditions that required treatment, and that they were likely to reoffend without close supervision. These courts were designed using a collaborative, rather than an adversarial, model. In an adversarial model, the state's attorney's primary duty is to protect public safety and to seek justice. In a collaborative model, both the state and the defense attorneys work for the goal of offender rehabilitation. In a collaborative model, the judge becomes the team leader, who monitors progress and provides rewards and sanctions. In an adversarial model, the judge is a neutral and an impartial decision maker, whose primary obligation is to uphold the law rather than rehabilitate the offender. The most common types of specialty courts are drug court and mental health court.

The first mental health courts were created in King's County, Washington, and Broward County, Florida, in the late 1990s. In 2000, Congress passed a law that provided funding for up to one hundred new mental health courts. They were modeled after the first specialty, or problem-oriented, court, the drug court, and were designed specifically to supervise and monitor chronically mentally ill misdemeanor offenders.

In addition to the judge and the attorneys involved in the case, mental health courts often involve the participation of social workers, probation agents, jail officials, and community treatment providers. The court acts as a liaison between community care providers and the correctional system by ensuring that the offender stays in treatment while in the community, and by providing clinical information to the jail when the offender is incarcerated.

Each mental health court has established criteria to determine eligibility for the program. In some jurisdictions, any DSM-IV diagnosis qualifies for inclusion, while in others, the defendant must have a psychotic illness, such as schizophrenia. Some jurisdictions allow defendants who primarily have a traumatic brain injury or developmental disability, while others bar this. The legal inclusion and exclusion criteria also vary. Most mental health courts will not accept defendants with a history of serious violent offenses such as rape or murder, and some courts refuse defendants with a history of simple assault.

Once a defendant is accepted to mental health court, he must sign a document that serves as the basis for the treatment contract. It outlines the specific treatment conditions the offender must agree to in order to remain in free society. Some courts require the defendant to plead guilty to his charge, in which case the treatment contract becomes a probation agreement. In other jurisdictions, the charge is automatically dropped or suspended prior to trial. In this case, the mental health court is a form of pretrial diversion back to the community. Since mental health court is voluntary, defendants can refuse the treatment contract. If this happens, the defendant is prosecuted through the regular court system.

Once the offender is released back to the community, the court schedules periodic hearings, known as status conferences, to monitor progress and compliance. These conferences are held in a courtroom in the presence of the treatment provider, jail representative, and legal counsel. A progress report is given to the judge, and the offender is given the opportunity to address the court and discuss his problems, or to explain issues related to noncompliance. The judge then provides feedback, either agreed-on rewards or agreed-on sanctions. The sanction may be removing the offender from the community for a brief period of incarceration. Finally, if all goes well, and the offender successfully completes his term of supervision, the court will hold a formal public graduation ceremony.

But does compelled treatment work?

Yes.

Preliminary outcome data have suggested that involvement in a mental health court reduces recidivism and use of inpatient services. Substance abuse programs welcome court supervision because the offender is more likely to show up for an intake appointment and to return for follow-up.

Despite documented success, mental health courts are not without controversy. While patient advocacy and professional organizations endorse the use of mental health courts because they divert patients out of the criminal justice system, critics of these courts allege that the use of incarceration as a sanction (that is, sending the defendant to jail for a period if he does not comply with the treatment plan) is an unconstitutional violation of due process. Although the defendant must sign a treatment agreement and must agree to participate in mental health court, critics also allege that the treatment provided is not truly voluntary. At least two states have filed class action suits challenging the constitutionality of specialty courts in general. Finally, there is also concern about the lack of confidentiality in mental health court programs, since information is shared freely between institutions and agencies and even discussed in public hearings.

The general issue of coercion in mental health care is an area of active research in psychiatry. The landmark study done on this topic was conducted by the MacArthur Foundation's research network on mental health and the law. This study showed that leveraged treatment is not necessarily perceived as coercive by the patient if the patient is given a chance to participate in the process, for example, by being included in the mental health status conference with the judge. In other words, coercion is in the eye of the beholder.

Since Eddie had both mental health and substance abuse problems, the judge agreed to place him on probation on the condition that he enroll in mental health court. Eddie was quick to agree, and he signed the treatment contract. He was released from the local jail and went to live with his grandmother Carolyn. Carolyn helped him set up an appointment at the local mental health clinic and paid for his medication. She provided transportation so that he could report to his probation officer and attend substance abuse therapy. For several months, he did well.

Then Carolyn had a stroke and was hospitalized. Without her supervision, Eddie fell apart. He reconnected with his "drug buddy" Bernie and relapsed. One night they broke into a convenience store intending to steal cash, cigarettes, and beer. Instead, they found a young woman locking up for the night. They forced her into the store and raped her at knife point. Police investigators took a still photo of the suspects from the convenience store's surveillance video and had it broadcast on the evening news. Within two days, Eddie was in police custody after an anonymous caller phoned a tip to the local police department. Police recovered cash and drugs from Carolyn's house.

Because Eddie was an adult, the police took him to the local jail. He went before a court commissioner and was denied bail. He was assigned a public defender, Jim Pringle, who visited him in jail.

The county jail was a decrepit building with imposing castlelike turrets. It had been in continuous use for over a hundred years and had few basic amenities. The housing tiers were too cold in the winter and too hot in the spring, and they smelled like dead mice. The visiting area was a small hallway with six whitewashed cement cubicles. Each cubicle contained a cracked plastic chair and a flat shield of Lexan glass that separated the visitor from the inmate. There was a small slot cut out of the shield that allowed papers to be slid back and forth. Eddie was escorted into the cubicle by a correctional officer, who held him by the back of his waist chain. His hands were shackled together and his leg irons made him walk with a short, shuffling gait. He was dressed in an orange jumpsuit that didn't fit.

"We need to be realistic here," said Eddie's lawyer. "They've got a video surveillance of the business. They've got your co-defendant implicating you, and it's just a matter of time before they get the DNA. I may be able to work a plea deal with the state since you've never been in trouble before as an adult, but you've got to give me something to work with."

"If they want me for the drugs, I'll take a CDS charge, but I ain't doin' no rape time," said Eddie. Mr. Pringle knew that Eddie was facing more than a misdemeanor charge for a controlled dangerous substance. He also knew that there was overwhelming evidence of his guilt, specifically a videotape of the crime. The best chance Eddie had for getting a plea deal was to take responsibility for his behavior.

In Eddie's case, there was conclusive evidence, and a judge or jury would likely find him guilty. Often, this is not the case, and evidence may be circumstantial or sketchy, so a confession is crucial to obtaining a conviction. But why would a criminal admit to doing something bad when there's little evidence to convict him? A more perplexing question is why someone might confess to a crime he *didn't* commit. To understand this, it's important to know something about the history of interrogation and about modern interrogation techniques.

Among the most infamous interrogators were the medieval inquisitors, church officials charged with the investigation of heresy. In the Middle Ages, the law was divided into secular law (the law of the king) and ecclesiastical, or church, law. Ecclesiastical law placed a heavy emphasis on confession as a means of absolution that would restore the offender into church society and into God's good graces. Failure to confess placed the offender at risk of eternal damnation. The inquisitors, who were responsible for both the heretic's soul and the preservation of church doctrine, were highly motivated to extract confessions. The chief interrogation techniques during this time involved physical torture such as the rack, the iron maiden, and thumbscrews. Water boarding, the interrogation technique made infamous at Guantanamo Bay prison, was also used in the Middle Ages. Not surprisingly, confessions were obtained easily.

Interrogation techniques began to change in 1215 following the adoption of the Magna Carta. This document limited the power of kings to detain people indefinitely, and it established the origin of the modern judicial system. It required a trial by a jury of one's peers and the use of independent judges. Modern criminal procedure expanded to include other rights for criminal defendants, such as the protection against self-incrimination. In other words, defendants could no longer be compelled to confess. Miranda warnings began as a way of preventing self-incrimination.

But criminals still confess.

The fact is that psychological interrogation techniques can be just as effective as physical torture for obtaining information. Modern investigators actually prefer psychological techniques because they are less likely to produce false information. Police investigators are legally allowed to use almost any means short of physical abuse to interrogate suspects. Interrogation has become a science and a topic of popular interest, to the extent that an Amazon.com book search on the term "police interrogation" will net over five thousand results.

Ironically similar to psychotherapy, modern interrogation involves a combination of personality and technique. The interrogator is someone skilled in the establishment of rapport. He tries to connect with the suspect and make him feel relaxed in the interrogation room by making small talk or offering food and a chance to smoke. Gradually the conversation works its way to the investigation of the crime. A skilled interrogator knows how to conduct and control an interview, how to collect information, and how to present it back to a suspect in a way that is designed to elicit more information. Reframing, rationalization, and altruistic appeals are examples of interviewing techniques.

The reframing technique means that the interrogator presents the circumstances of the offense to the suspect in a way that makes it psychologically easier to admit involvement, for example, by telling the suspect, "Witness X says you did this, but I'm sure it didn't happen the way X said it did. I doubt it was that bad. It was an accident, or no one meant it to end up that way." Reframing is also used to change the way the suspect views his own involvement, for example, by suggesting, "You're not evil. What you did wasn't evil. You're just sick and need help. The best way to get help is to tell me what happened." The rationalization technique involves the offer of excuses: "Victim Y was a nasty old son-of-a-gun, and he had it coming. It was bound to happen. I'd like to shake the hand of whoever did him in." Finally, altruistic appeals are a way of inducing the suspect to offer information to protect real or false alternative suspects: "We know your wife [or girlfriend or mother] was involved, but we won't charge them if you give yourself up." Outright lies are also legally allowed, the most common one being "We know you did it. We just need you to fill in the details."

While investigators are trained and skilled, criminal suspects are not. They generally have bad judgment or may be immature or mentally ill.

They might be in drug or alcohol withdrawal at the time of the interrogation. Developmentally disabled suspects may feel a need to please the investigator by giving the information they think police are looking for. A suspect's personality traits can make him susceptible to certain techniques. Someone with a need for admiration may be flattered to induce him to brag about his crimes. All these factors can lower resistance to questioning.

Finally, some criminals confess for a simple and obvious reason: they feel guilty, and it's the "right" thing to do. For these folks, confession is a means of absolution in the historical, religious sense of the term, and it can be a relief.

Eddie wasn't sold on the idea of a confession. "You're supposed to be helping me, right? Why don't you tell the judge everything I need help with? Maybe I can go back to mental health court." He told his lawyer everything that he hoped would lead to a more lenient outcome: the loss of his mother to AIDS, his unstable early home life, his grandmother's illness, his drug use, his history of mental health treatment.

"You've seen a psychiatrist?" Mr. Pringle asked. "Have you been treated with medication?"

"Yeah," said Eddie. "A lot of them. They gave me depression medicine, medicine for ADHD, and medicine to help me with my temper. None of it really worked. Finally, I just gave up and quit going."

"That's important to know. I'll want the judge to know more about that too." Mr. Pringle went on to explain that he was going to ask the judge to order an examination of Eddie's competence to stand trial, and that he was also going to file an insanity plea on Eddie's behalf.

"But I'm not crazy!" Eddie exclaimed.

"Since I know about your psychiatric history, as your attorney I have a duty to represent you the best I can. The judge has to know that you're mentally OK to participate in your trial. And I need to know if there's any basis to go forward with an insanity defense. Just talk to the court psychiatrist," Mr. Pringle said. When Eddie was taken to bail review, the judge agreed that a pretrial psychiatric evaluation was needed. She signed the order for the evaluation, and two weeks later Eddie was transported from the jail to the courthouse to see the doctor.

There he met a forensic psychiatrist named Dr. Sam Huber. Pictures of hunting dogs hung on the walls of his office, and a sculpture of a pheasant sat on a small credenza.

Dr. Huber took Eddie's history and asked many questions about the offense. He asked questions about Eddie's use of alcohol and drugs at the time of the crime and about his motives for committing the rape. He asked a lot of questions about Eddie's sex life, which Eddie found embarrassing, but he went along with the questions on the advice of his lawyer. Dr. Huber asked a lot of detailed questions about the psychiatric symptoms Eddie had experienced in the past and about the presence of any symptoms at the time of the crime. The interview was longer and more detailed than any interview Eddie had ever had with a psychiatrist. Finally, after four hours of questions, Dr. Huber told Eddie what he thought about the insanity defense.

"Well, I need to review your treatment records and talk to your family, but from what you've told me so far, you were in pretty good contact with reality at the time the crime happened. You weren't hearing voices or having delusions. In fact, that has never been an issue for you. You and your friend had been drinking a bit, and the cocaine probably didn't help either. You don't have much in the way of an insanity defense."

This response didn't surprise Eddie. He had told his lawyer he wasn't crazy. But he did want to know what was wrong with him. Here he was, at age 18, facing a long prison sentence. Normal people just didn't do things like this.

"Doc, can you tell me what's wrong with me? Why do I keep getting in trouble over and over again?"

This seems like an odd question with an obvious answer. It would be easy to say that Eddie kept getting in trouble simply because he was a criminal, but there is a difference between someone who has been convicted of a single crime and someone with a pattern of criminal behavior. Repetitive criminals may be psychopaths or sociopaths.

We have known about psychopaths for a long time. In 1837, an English psychiatrist named James Pritchard wrote a book entitled *Treatise on Insanity* in which he described people who lacked the ability to form attachments to others and who were unable to experience normal human affection or emotions. These individuals had little regard for the feelings or rights of others; however, they didn't have the hallucinations or impaired cognitive functioning that was seen in other psychiatric disorders. Dr. Pritchard coined the term *moral insanity* to describe this disorder, which he felt was a defect in the area of the brain responsible for moral reasoning. Around this time, the *American Journal of Insanity* (which later became the *American Journal of Psychiatry*) published several individual case studies of homicide offenders, all of which were entitled "A Case of Homicidal Insanity." They were all essentially just case descriptions of murderers. The letters to the editor of the journal following these case studies debated the validity of moral insanity as a mental illness. The term insanity was controversial because it implied that from a legal standpoint, the criminal should not be held responsible or punished for his behavior. Eventually the term moral insanity was dropped in favor of psychopath, a term proposed by a nineteenth-century German psychiatrist, J. L. Koch.

More recently, the term sociopath has been used instead of psychopath. This latest change happened because people were getting confused by the "psycho" part of the psychopathy label—psychopathy doesn't mean that the criminal is psychotic. Actually, neither sociopathy nor psychopathy are official psychiatric diagnoses in the *Diagnostic and Statistical Manual* (DSM). The DSM uses the term antisocial personality disorder (ASPD). Patients with ASPD are known for lying, repeated criminal acts, and impulsivity or irresponsibility. The majority of people with ASPD are not psychopaths. Psychopaths represent a minority of severely disordered people who lack emotional attachments or responsiveness. They are narcissistic and are unable to learn from experience. They lack empathy or remorse and are cold, cruel, callous people. This callousness is what distinguishes psychopathy from antisocial personality disorder.

A lot of people have ASPD—about 3 percent of the United States population, or 9 million people. On the other hand, the exact prevalence of psychopathy may never be known because psychopaths usually come to the attention of clinicians only when they are caught committing crimes or when those around them coerce them into treatment. Not everyone who has a disregard for consequences and an inability to empathize with others becomes a violent criminal, however. Some people with these characteristics function successfully as politicians, religious leaders, or heads of large corporations and come to public attention only if they get caught breaking a law.

A screening tool for psychopathy developed in the 1980s has been widely used in research and forensic practice. Scores on the Hare Psychopathy Check List–Revised (PCL-R) have been useful for predicting violence and criminal recidivism. Scientists are using psychopaths identified by the PCL-R to study the physical basis for the disorder. They've found that psychopaths' emotional reactions are different from other people, and they don't show the normal physiologic responses to fear: increased heart rate, increased blood pressure, and moist skin. Functional neuroimaging can also be used to show that psychopaths process emotional reactions differently. Functional neuroimaging studies measure changes in blood flow to different parts of the brain, and this in turn is a measure of the brain's activity level. When psychopaths are shown violent or frightening pictures, there is less activity in the parts of the brain that regulate emotions compared with normal people.

There is a genetic component to both ASPD and psychopathy, as shown by adoption and twin studies. Some twin studies have shown that for severe psychopaths, as much as two-thirds of psychopathy can be attributed to genetics rather than environmental influences. For ASPD, the condition originates in childhood. A study done in the 1960s followed children from a mental health center who were referred for evaluation of their behavior problems. The study found that fifteen years later, one-third of the children with conduct disorder grew up to have antisocial personality disorder.

Can psychopaths be treated?

This is a tough question to answer. Psychopaths don't seek treatment voluntarily because they aren't bothered by their condition. They must be coerced into treatment or persuaded to participate by having their self-interest engaged, for example, if treatment is a condition of parole and is necessary to stay out of jail or prison. Since psychopaths have difficulty learning from consequences, several treatment attempts may be necessary. The treatment must be designed to have open lines of communication with others to ensure truthfulness. There must be clear, consistent, and firm boundaries between the patient and the therapist. Psychopaths with a high risk of violent behavior need to be treated in a secure and structured setting, like a correctional facility. Psychopaths and people with ASPD are at increased risk of developing other psychiatric conditions such as mood disorders and substance abuse. Medication is used for treatment of these coexisting conditions.

There is no evidence that psychopathy or ASPD can be cured. The goal of treatment is to minimize the impact of the conditions on others and on the patient. For example, one goal of treatment might be to minimize the risk of accidental injury by teaching the patient to recognize situations that trigger dangerous risk-taking behavior. Violence is another focus of treatment with psychopaths; violent behavior can be managed with administrative disciplinary procedures within the correctional facility. Medication may be helpful. Specific treatment goals should be set up collaboratively with the patient so that expectations and treatment parameters are clear.

"So I've got a mental problem called antisocial personality? If I've got a problem, why wouldn't I be insane?" Eddie asked hopefully. By now he realized that he was not going to escape a prison term for rape, and the insanity defense was sounding more and more appealing.

Dr. Huber explained that just having a mental disorder was not enough to meet the legal criteria for insanity.

"In order to be legally insane, you have to have some connection between the mental disorder and the crime," he said. "There must be some evidence that the mental illness affected your ability to understand what you were doing, or that what you were doing was wrong. People with antisocial personality disorder do have the ability to know when their behavior is criminal."

The state has to prove two issues to convict a defendant. First, the state must prove that the defendant actually committed the crime—that he pulled the trigger or stabbed the victim. In legal language, this issue is known as the *actus reus,* or criminal act. Next, the state must prove that the defendant meant to commit the crime when he did the act. In other words, that the behavior was not a mere accident or unexpected result. For example, if someone accidentally started a forest fire by dropping a match while lighting a cigarette, this would not be arson because the defendant didn't have the required criminal intent or guilty mental state. In legal language the criminal intent or mental state is known as the *mens rea*. If the defense can create reasonable doubt about either the defendant's actus reus or his mens rea, the defendant will be acquitted of the crime, or convicted of a less serious offense.

Many legal defense strategies are based on the idea that the defendant wasn't in the right state of mind at the time of the crime. A defense attorney might argue that the defendant was acting in a jealous rage, under the influence of some hallucinogenic drug, or in fear for his life. These defenses are all known as mens rea defenses. The insanity defense is another type of mens rea defense.

Insanity defenses are usually filed on behalf of defendants who have psychotic illnesses, such as schizophrenia, but it's possible to use disorders other than those found in the DSM-IV. For example, battered spouse syndrome is not a DSM diagnosis, but it has been used as the basis for an insanity plea. By law, either the judge or the jury decides if a given disorder "counts" as a mental disease.

The decision to pursue an insanity defense is usually made on strategic rather than clinical grounds. Lots of criminal defendants have histories of mental illness, but very few rely on this defense because most mentally ill defendants are accused of minor crimes. Misdemeanor offenders typically serve only months in jail if they're convicted, but an insanity acquittee could be institutionalized in a hospital indefinitely if the plea is successful. Even after discharge, acquittees are sometimes supervised by the court for years. The defense attorney's responsibility is to secure the best possible outcome for his client. Thus, the insanity plea is usually employed only when the defendant is charged with a felony.

When the case goes to trial, the judge or jury must look at the evidence and decide if the facts of the case meet the legal standard for insanity. This standard, also known as the insanity test, has developed through case law and legislation over the last 150 years. Each state has some variation of this defense except for Montana, Kansas, Utah, and Idaho, which have abolished it.

Historically, there have been four main legal tests for insanity, and most states use a variation of three of them: the McNaughten test, the irresistible impulse test, the product test (also sometimes called the Durham rule), and the Model Penal Code, or American Law Institute (ALI) test.

The *McNaughten test* was created in the nineteenth century, in Britain, following an infamous case in which a mentally ill man tried to assassinate the British prime minister. He was found insane, and the outrage following the verdict lead the House of Lords to order the creation of the first legal standard for insanity. The McNaughten test says that a defendant is insane if he is unable to appreciate the wrongfulness of his actions. The *irresistible impulse test* was developed later in the nineteenth century. This test says that a defendant is insane if he was overcome by the strength of the mental illness to the extent that he couldn't control his behavior or refrain from committing the crime. The *product test*, or *Durham rule*, was created in the 1950s as a result of greater understanding of mental illness. The court wanted a looser test out of recognition that many mental illnesses did not affect the ability to understand actions, but did affect judgment. The Durham rule states that a defendant is insane if the crime was the result of a mental illness. This standard was eventually rejected as being too loose. Finally, in the 1970s the ALI created the *Model Penal Code* in an attempt to make criminal laws more uniform among states. The ALI test states that a defendant is insane if he is unable to appreciate the criminality of his conduct or to conform his conduct to the requirements of the law. The ALI test combines the cognitive insanity standard of the McNaughten test with the volitional or behavioral standard of the irresistible impulse test.

Following a successful insanity defense, the defendant (now known as an acquittee) is committed to a hospital for treatment. Insanity acquittees don't get placed in regular psychiatric hospitals. They go to forensic hospitals, inpatient units designed to treat people who are violent as a result of mental illness. Forensic hospitals are unique because of their focus on security in addition to treatment. Inpatient units in forensic hospitals have security technicians, or aides, who provide physical protection to staff and patients. They also have specific entry and exit procedures to control the flow of contraband into the facility. Forensic hospitals typically have policies for regular searches of the inpatient units, or of the patients themselves, to prevent weapons from entering the hospital.

Unlike nonforensic, or civil, patients, insanity acquittees may be hospitalized for years. By law, acquittees can be committed until they are either no longer mentally ill or no longer dangerous. They have the option of requesting discharge or a review of their commitment periodically. This review is usually done by the judge who committed the patient, although some states allow a jury to review the commitment through a process known as a conditional release hearing.

When the acquittee is ready to be discharged, he is placed on conditional release. This means that he is allowed to leave the hospital, with the court's approval, only if he agrees to abide by certain conditions. Many of these conditions are similar to those found in a parole agreement—refrain from committing new crimes and avoid abuse of drugs or alcohol. Some conditions are specific to the acquittee, such as requirements to take psychiatric medication and to keep therapy appointments. The length of time for conditional release varies among states but is usually about five years with options for incremental renewal. If the acquittee fails to keep his appointments or take medication, he can be picked up by police and brought back to the hospital.

Eddie's lawyer decided there was no reason to pursue the insanity plea once he read Dr. Huber's report. And once the lab report came back confirming the DNA evidence, Eddie realized a plea deal was his only option. When the state's attorney approached Mr. Pringle with a five-year deal for a third-degree sex offense rather than a rape, Eddie agreed to plead guilty. Because of Eddie's age, the judge accepted the plea and sentenced him to the time recommended by the prosecutor. Two days after his court appearance, Eddie was transferred from the jail to the state prison system.

Up to now, Eddie had been a pretrial detainee, someone charged with a crime but not convicted. Pretrial detainees are presumed to be innocent and have some rights that are not available to convicted criminals. Once he was found guilty and sentenced, Eddie became a convicted criminal, even worse, a convicted sex offender. Convicted criminals are held in prison rather than in jail. Jail is where someone waits to go to trial; prison is where a criminal goes to serve his sentence.

Eddie was sent first to a reception center, a specialized type of prison where convicts are housed temporarily while awaiting assignment to a permanent facility. In the reception center, he was assigned to a security level through a process known as classification. Because it was his first time through the Division of Correction, he was assigned to medium security. At the reception center, he also went through a screening process to see if he had any medical or psychiatric conditions that required treatment. A physician's assistant read him questions from a form about various diseases and symptoms and about his history of psychiatric care. Because Eddie had received psychiatric medications in the past, he was automatically referred to the institution's psychiatrist.

The reception center was newer than the jail Eddie had been in, meaning that it was only 45 years old. The ventilation system worked, and the elevators also usually worked, but on the day that Eddie was sent to see the prison psychiatrist, the elevators weren't working, so he was escorted along with a group of nine other inmates down three flights of stairs and through the long hallway leading to the psychology department. Eddie glanced into the rooms he walked by and saw people trying to work in an uncomfortable environment. There were wastebaskets in the middle of the hallway and inside a couple of offices, perched to catch the water dripping from the ceiling. Broken pipes were everywhere. Just as the smell of mildew was becoming overwhelming, he was told to step through the open office door of Dr. Larry Vitti.

Dr. Vitti's office was unlike any psychiatrist's office that Eddie had ever been in. There was no comfortable sofa, no framed artwork or diplomas on the walls, no window with a nice view of the outdoors, no plants, not even a carpet. Dr. Vitti was working in what appeared to be an old unused prison cell. There was a stainless steel toilet in a corner of the room, but the sink had been removed, leaving exposed pipes. The transporting officer told Eddie to sit on one of the two folding chairs in the room. Dr. Vitti sat in the other, balancing a clipboard on his knees. He had no desk and no telephone.

"Hello, Mr. Banks," said Dr. Vitti. "Make yourself comfortable there, and I'll explain what's going on."

Eddie wasn't sure how anyone could make himself comfortable in a place like this. He also wondered what Dr. Vitti must have done wrong in the past, to lead him to work in a prison.

"I'm seeing you today because the medical department sent you down. The referral says you've had some mental health care in the past." Dr. Vitti reviewed Eddie's history with him and verified the details of his out-patient treatment and responses to medications.

"How are you doing today?" he asked.

"Not too good," said Eddie. "I'm not sleeping, my mind is racing all the time, and I feel like I'm going to flip out." He didn't want to admit it, but he also felt like crying much of the time. It wasn't a good idea to cry in prison, at least not where another inmate could see you.

Eddie was referred to the psychiatrist because he was identified through an intake screening process. Other inmates are referred by custody or by civilian prison staff, such as social workers or case managers, after intake. The symptoms that trigger these later referrals include aggressive or violent behavior, sexually inappropriate behavior, or disorganized and bizarre behavior like swallowing foreign objects or smearing feces on the walls of the cell. Inmates can also be referred for assessment of mental status changes such as confusion or disorientation. Also, inmates have the option of requesting mental health care at any point in an incarceration.

The symptoms Eddie described were very familiar to Dr. Vitti. Many newly incarcerated inmates report insomnia, anxiety, sadness, and concentration difficulties, particularly during a first incarceration. Most initial symptoms resolve within two weeks. The main challenge for a forensic psychiatrist in a correctional facility is to differentiate between temporary adjustment symptoms and the more serious condition of clinical depression. The symptoms of depression are more difficult to interpret when the patient is a prisoner. For example, one symptom of clinical depression is excessive or inappropriate guilt. How can a psychiatrist decide exactly how much guilt is "inappropriate or excessive" for a murderer? Another symptom of major depression is insomnia. In correctional settings, insomnia is present in most prisoners regardless of their psychiatric status. It's just not a reliable diagnostic symptom.

A prisoner with clinical depression will typically have persistent feelings of sadness beyond the usual two- or three-week initial adjustment period. The low mood is accompanied by loss of motivation or interest in recreation. The clinically depressed inmate will report that he doesn't come out of his cell for recreation, that he has lost interest in exercising in his cell, that he doesn't feel like socializing or talking to other inmates, and that he has difficulty concentrating to read books or write letters to his family. Clinically depressed inmates also often report decreased frustration tolerance and a shorter temper than usual. This is the symptom that will often prompt an inmate to seek mental health care in prison, even if he's never had treatment before. Prisoners fear loss of control or fighting because they could be placed in disciplinary lockdown or segregated housing for a rule infraction. This would also lead to loss of visiting and recreation privileges.

Dr. Vitti talked to Eddie about his symptoms and explained that the way he was feeling was part of the normal institutional adjustment process. Eddie agreed to come back for a follow-up appointment two or three weeks later to make sure his symptoms were resolving. Dr. Vitti knew that Eddie had been treated for depression in the past, so he explained that Eddie could receive mental health services at any facility he was sent to during his incarceration. "In fact," he added. "I work at another prison near here, so if you get transferred to that facility, I may see you again."

"Can they get me back on Paxil if I need it later?" Eddie asked. "That's what I took before, on the outside."

Medication decisions are more complicated for forensic psychiatrists in correctional facilities than for psychiatrists in free society. This is because correctional psychiatrists have an obligation to consider the impact of their prescribing practices on the correctional health care system as well as on the institution. Each correctional health care system is given a limited annual budget but a potentially unlimited number of patients. The use of expensive new medications will affect the number of patients that can be treated. Older, cheaper, and equally effective medications are often preferred in correctional systems. Many public health care systems rely on medication formularies, or standard medication lists, that clinicians must adhere to.

Correctional psychiatrists must also keep in mind that any medication prescribed for one patient may fall into the hands of another, particularly medications with sedating side effects, which have significant value in the prison micro-economy. Vulnerable inmates may be intimidated into giving up their sedating medications to their peers.

There are many valid clinical reasons for changing the medications a prisoner was taking in free society, and these reasons have nothing to do with health care costs or systemwide policies. Medication needs change depending on the environment. For example, a prisoner with diabetes will need less insulin in prison because he'll be getting a controlled diabetic diet and will have limited access to off-diet foods. Some prisoners will need less (and sometimes no) psychiatric medication once they are abstinent from drugs and alcohol in a controlled environment. Sometimes the free society treatment has been prescribed by a nonpsychiatrist and is not consistent with recommended standards. There are too many hypothetical possibilities to cover them all, but those are the most common reasons correctional psychiatrists prescribe medications that are different from those a prisoner received in free society.

About three weeks after Eddie saw Dr. Vitti, he was transferred to his maintaining facility, the prison where he was assigned to serve his time. Over the course of the next year, he got his GED, stayed out of trouble, and got a job as a cook in the prison kitchen. By the end of his first year of incarceration, he was eligible to have his security status lowered to minimum security through a process called reclassification. He saw a case manager who reviewed his prison base file, including records of his prison disciplinary history and participation in jobs and classes. Eddie had had no rule infractions or disciplinary issues, and his adjustment history was good. The case manager was inclined to agree with the lower security status, but because Eddie was a sex offender, and minimum security inmates are sometimes allowed out of the facility to work, he wanted a risk evaluation and recommendations from the institutional psychology department. Eddie was sent back to see Dr. Vitti.

"It's been a long time since I've seen you, Mr. Banks," said Dr. Vitti. "I hope that means you've been doing OK?"

"I have, doc. Trust me, you'd hear from me if I weren't. Everybody around here says you actually care about what happens to people here. I'd drop a note if I were having trouble." Eddie looked very different than he had when he'd first come to prison. He had regained the weight he'd lost while using cocaine. He was clean shaven and had a neat haircut. His attitude was different too. He had accomplishments under his belt that he was proud of. He told Dr. Vitti about his grandmother Carolyn, who was finally home after suffering a stroke. He talked about getting his GED and about getting accepted into (and completing) the institutional home improvement program as well as the substance abuse relapse prevention program. He showed Dr. Vitti his program certificates.

"I did all this," he said. "All I need from you is something saying I'm OK for minimum security."

"I'll be frank with you, Mr. Banks," said Dr. Vitti. "Everything you've done is terrific, but the fact that you're a convicted sex offender means that there's no guarantee you'll get to minimum. One of the reasons you were referred here is to do a risk assessment, in other words, to give some input to case management about the likelihood that you'll commit another rape."

Eddie was shocked. "That ain't *ever* gonna happen again!" he exclaimed. "I was drunk, I was high, I did something stupid. I'm not a rapist."

"I know the details of your case, but in addition to that, I'm going to have the prison psychologist see you, too, to do some tests. The psychologist will talk to you and send some recommendations on to case management. What you also need to be aware of is that in this state, there is a sex offender commitment law. This means that at the end of your time, there's a chance that the state may try to send you to a psychiatric hospital."

Eddie was excited. "You mean I could go somewhere for treatment?" he said. "Why wait until my time is over? Can I go there now?"

"No, you don't understand," said Dr. Vitti. "You'd get sent to a hospital *after* you've served your time in prison, through something called a civil commitment. A civil commitment is where a judge orders you to stay in a hospital. For sex offenders, once you've been committed, there's no guarantee you'll ever get out."

In the 1950s some states created therapeutic prisons, facilities designed specifically around a therapeutic model. Offenders were offered group and individual therapy and were released only when a team of mental health professionals decided they were ready for parole. States also passed laws, known as *defective delinquent* statutes, that would allow for indefinite commitment of violent criminals to psychiatric hospitals for treatment. One of the earliest commitment laws for criminals was adopted in Minnesota in 1939. It was known as the psychopathic personality statute, and it allowed for commitment of people who suffered from "conditions of emotional instability, or impulsiveness of behavior, or lack of customary standards of good judgment, or failure to appreciate the consequences of his acts, or a combination of any such conditions, as to render such person irresponsible for his conduct with respect to sexual matters and thereby dangerous to other persons."

If an offender met criteria for being a psychopathic personality, he was committed "for the rest of his life to an asylum for the dangerously insane." The statute was promptly and unsuccessfully challenged as unconstitutionally vague and a violation of equal protection in the 1940 case *Pearson v. Probate*. Pearson alleged that the definition of a psychopathic personality was too broad and that people who weren't psychopathic could be committed by mistake. The United States Supreme Court acknowledged that there was a risk of abuse in the statute and that it could be used for political ends; however, the Court concluded that the existing commitment procedures were adequate to protect the offenders' rights.

Today, seventeen states have laws that allow the indefinite commitment of sex offenders. The construction of the laws vary considerably regarding who makes the release decision and the standard of proof for commitment. Over the last ten years, several legal cases have challenged various aspects of the commitment process.

In 1997 the United States Supreme Court decided *Kansas v. Hendricks*. Hendricks was an admitted pedophile who was scheduled to be released from prison. He was civilly committed under the state's Sexually Violent Predator Act, which allowed for commitment of people with mental abnormalities or personality disorders who were "likely to engage in predatory acts of sexual violence." Hendricks appealed his commitment, alleging that it should have been based on "mental illness" rather than "mental abnormality." He also made a claim of double jeopardy, that he was being given a second punishment for a single crime. He lost on both counts. The Supreme Court said that it would leave the states to determine their own definition of mental illness, and that a civil commitment could not be considered a second punishment because the purpose was for treatment.

Within three months of the Hendricks decision, the National Association of State Mental Health Program Directors adopted a position statement objecting to it. They did not acknowledge sexual paraphilias as a legitimate diagnosable mental illness and objected to the idea that the commitment was for the purpose of treatment. Clearly, sex offenders were not welcome in psychiatric hospitals.

The follow-up to Hendricks came in the 2002 case *Kansas v. Crane*. Crane was a committed exhibitionist who challenged his institutionalization because the judge at his commitment hearing did not make any finding about him being unable to control his dangerous behavior. Traditional commitment laws require that the patient be both mentally ill and dangerous. The Sexually Violent Predator Act required that the dangerousness be based on a "difficulty or inability to control" the dangerous behavior. The Kansas Supreme Court overturned his commitment because the trial judge never said Crane was unable to control his behavior. The U.S. Supreme Court found that this interpretation of the statute was overly strict—that it was enough just to show the patient had difficulty or impairment in his behavioral control. After this case, courts had to prove a volitional element during the civil commitment hearings, in addition to proving that a mental abnormality existed.

In states with civil commitment laws, over one thousand sex offenders have been confined to psychiatric hospitals after they've served their prison sentences. Only a handful have ever been released, making the efficacy of sex offender commitment difficult to assess. While public safety is one justification for commitment, as yet we have little evidence that sex offenses are reduced in states that have offender commitment laws. Costs for treating sex offenders range from $30,000 to $125,000 per inmate per year, and the cost for running a secure facility for committed offenders was $214 million annually in 2005. Committed sex offenders are requiring more of each state's budget, at a time when there are fewer resources available to those with mental illness who have not committed crimes.

The costs of sex offender commitment programs are going to rise because advocacy organizations are now challenging the adequacy of the treatment given in these facilities and their environmental conditions.

Litigation costs, and the cost of improved services, are an additional financial burden.

Sex offender commitment laws are expensive and lack proven effects on public safety. They consume resources intended for those with serious psychotic illnesses. As states trend away from commitment policies, they will likely continue to pursue other options such as enhanced criminal sentences, sex offender registries, mandatory reporting laws, and extended home monitoring programs.

What happened to Eddie? He had a hard start in life and followed the path he seemed destined for, ending in prison. While in prison, he made several changes with the hope of starting a new, more responsible life. Fortunately, both the psychology department and the case management reports were favorable. Eddie Banks was transferred to a minimum security prison and successfully transitioned to work release eighteen months later. He was not considered for indefinite commitment because the psychology report documented that he was a low risk for recidivism. Finally, he was released on parole. Because he was a convicted sex offender, he had to follow several standard conditions. He had to report to the local police station upon release and keep them notified of his current address. He was also barred from living within 1,000 feet of any school and from having unsupervised contact with children, even though his only offense was against an adult. Fortunately, Carolyn did not live near a school. Eddie did well at his work release job as an electrician. His employer kept him on after release, and he used his salary to help care for his grandmother. Mental health care was also a condition of his parole, and he found it helpful to have a therapist he could talk to when he felt stressed. By the time his parole ended, he stayed in treatment because by then he knew he needed it, and it helped.

There are many people like Eddie in the prisons of this country, some with violent histories but most with less serious issues. Whether or not they get a chance at a new life is up to society and the laws we create.

Chapter 9

Mitchell:
Hospital-based Psychiatry

MITCHELL'S MOTHER started to worry when he was a sophomore in high school. He stopped going out with friends, he lost interest in sports, and he only came out of his room when he had to. Nothing much interested him, but he insisted he was fine. Mitchell's father thought this was a phase and said his wife was a worrier who was overreacting. It became a struggle to get Mitchell to shower, shave, or wear deodorant, and he seemed oblivious to the things teenagers usually care about. At the end of Mitchell's senior year, it became clear that something was terribly wrong. Mitchell started hearing soft, whispering voices and believed that people were conspiring against him. He had hallucinations and delusions, and his mother was afraid that he suffered from schizophrenia, just like her younger brother. Mitchell had completely lost contact with reality and everyone agreed that he needed to be in the hospital where he could get help.

In the previous chapters, we've talked about psychiatry as it pertains to outpatient and forensic settings. Hospital-based psychiatry is mostly oriented to emergency and inpatient settings. In this chapter, we discuss different aspects of care that are rendered inside the hospital, looking at the process as Mitchell goes from the Emergency Department to the inpatient unit, to partial hospitalization, and then to the medical floors. We also talk about communication among the health care team and the use of electronic health records to improve care.

Hospital emergency rooms are where people go when they are too sick or too poor to go to a doctor's office, or when the office is closed and they cannot wait. Of course, these are no longer just emergency *rooms* but entire emergency *departments*. In fact, the term ED is now used more than ER by hospitals.

The ED is the entry point to the hospital for most people; 80 to 90 percent of hospital admissions begin in the ED for most hospitals. Patients go to the ED with any number of psychiatric problems, including panic attacks, suicidal feelings, depression, or drug or alcohol intoxication or withdrawal. Sometimes people arrive with an altered mental state, meaning they are confused or having memory problems. Mitchell came to the ED at his mother's insistence because he was hearing voices and was paranoid.

Some people are brought to the ED against their will, typically by the police, because someone's safety is in jeopardy. Most states have a law that provides for an emergency evaluation—in Maryland this is called an emergency petition (EP)—which gives police the authority to take someone to an ED for evaluation. Although judges can authorize an emergency evaluation that is triggered by a concerned citizen, most states permit a police officer or licensed health professional to execute an EP without a judge's intervention. There has to be some evidence of a mental illness in addition to behavior that is considered dangerous in some manner. In chapter 2, for example, Josh was brought to the ED on an emergency petition by the police after he threatened his roommate with a knife. A smaller number of states have outpatient commitment laws, which permit police to bring someone to the ED if they fail to follow through with required treatment.

One of the challenges of psychiatry is to balance societal safety with the individual's fundamental rights. Both legal and ethical considerations dictate elements of clinical practice. It is a difficult position to be in to have to commit someone to a hospital who crosses the threshold of being ill and unable to make good decisions. We struggle with where to draw that line, which is sometimes very fuzzy, to the point where these challenges will sometimes even find themselves intruding into our dreams. When the decision is particularly unclear, we will often call a colleague to further discuss the case.

Mitchell said very little to the triage nurse. She took his blood pressure and pulse, and Mitchell was sent to wait. He was seen briefly by the ED doctor, who asked a few questions and listened to Mitchell's heart and lungs.

"Does anything hurt?" the doctor asked Mitchell.

"What are those cameras for?" Mitchell asked.

"They're security cameras," the doctor answered. "Well, you look good," he said when he finished the exam. He spoke briefly to Mitchell's mother and told her a social worker would be in soon to see them. A technician drew Mitchell's blood, and Mitchell also provided a urine sample.

When someone comes to the ED, or is brought by emergency petition, the first doctor they see is typically not a psychiatrist but a physician who specializes in emergency medicine. She is the physician ultimately responsible for making the decisions about what treatment is recommended. After the interview, exam, and review of the relevant laboratory studies, the Emergency Department physician decides whether to recommend admission, unless she feels more information or expertise is needed. In that case, she requests a consult from a mental health professional to evaluate the patient in the ED. This person is often a clinical social worker, less frequently a psychiatric physician. If that clinician has sufficient concerns about either safety or liability, he may specifically request a consult from a psychiatrist, but many hospitals do not have 24/7 availability of psychiatrists in the ED. Hospitals that make psychiatrists available in the ED tend to hospitalize a lower proportion of patients since the psychiatrist has expertise in managing more complex situations. A physician without that expertise might simply make the decision to admit and let the inpatient unit figure out the best plan.

After the decision is made to admit a patient to a psychiatric unit, the next decision is about where to admit him. There are generally four options here: (1) admit to a psychiatric unit in the same hospital; (2) transfer to a psychiatric unit in another general hospital; (3) transfer to a free-standing psychiatric hospital; or (4) transfer to a state psychiatric hospital. This last option is becoming increasingly unavailable as expensive-to-maintain state hospitals close down or shrink in size. State psychiatric hospitals are also increasingly occupied by forensic patients who are held there by the courts, leaving fewer beds available for patients who aren't involved in the criminal justice system.

What determines whether a patient gets admitted to a psychiatric unit in the same hospital where he was initially seen or is sent elsewhere? Not all hospitals have psychiatric units. If the hospital has one, then admission will depend on whether it is already full, whether it treats patients with that age and condition, and whether its *acuity level* can accommodate a particular individual. If there are already four manic patients on a fifteen-bed unit, the hospital may not be able to safely accommodate a fifth, even if it has empty beds—it needs sufficient staff to supervise these more ill patients.

Mitchell told the social worker that he was hearing voices and that he felt scared. He was almost certain there were cameras in his house and that authorities were monitoring him, though he wasn't sure why. He talked about how he left a glass of water on his desk, and when he came back in the room, it was in a different position.

"What does that mean?" the social worker asked.

"You already know," Mitchell said. He seemed to think everyone was in on some type of plot. His mother said that sometimes she would hear Mitchell in the midst of a very animated conversation when he was alone in his room. He didn't have a good grasp of what was real, and sometimes his family was afraid of him because they didn't understand what was going on in his mind.

Mitchell agreed to enter the hospital voluntarily. The only problem was that all the psychiatric beds were full, and he would need to go to another hospital. The social worker said she would find him a bed. Mitchell's mother wanted him to be close to home so that family could visit; they had only one car and inflexible work schedules.

"I'll try," the social worker said. "Your insurance pays for beds only at certain facilities. It would actually be easier to find Mitchell a bed if he didn't have health insurance!"

Federal laws prevent transferring a patient with unstable medical or psychiatric conditions from an ED to another hospital solely for insurance reasons. A federal law called the Emergency Medical Treatment and Labor

Act (EMTALA) was enacted in 1986—though the regulations were not put into effect until 1994—to prevent instances of so-called patient dumping, when an uninsured patient is transferred to another hospital to avoid the costs of treating someone who cannot or will not pay. EMTALA requires that the patient be stabilized prior to transfer and that a physician at the receiving hospital authorize the transfer if the hospital possesses the capacity and capability to treat the patient. If the initial hospital lacks the capacity *or* capability to treat the patient, and another hospital has both, then that hospital *must* accept the patient regardless of the patient's ability to pay (or insurance authorization), or risk an EMTALA violation. A violation can cost a hospital up to $50,000 per infraction, so such violations are actively avoided in the hospital business.

In Mitchell's case, the hospital's psychiatric unit was full, so the ED social worker began the arduous process of performing a bed search. This often takes a long time and is one of the reasons patients requiring psychiatric hospitalization are often stuck in the ED for many hours, and sometimes days.

Most states do not have a central bed registry where one can call a single number, find out who has beds and what type, send the clinical information, and receive an acceptance. Such a mechanism would greatly improve this inefficient process. Instead, ED staff members call each hospital on their list to ask about bed availability. Typically, they leave a message, and the hospital calls back later. If a bed is available, the next step is to send the clinical information. Even in this era of electronic communication and with the push for hospitals to adopt electronic medical records, this clinical information is usually sent via fax. Sometimes the fax isn't received, or the machine is out of paper or gets jammed, causing more delays. The nurse reviews the information, shares it with the on-call psychiatrist, and this other hospital decides whether to accept the admission or not, based on the patient's appropriateness for that unit and the unit's acuity level. It sometimes takes several hours for a hospital to confirm that a bed is available, and then several more hours to get a decision on acceptance. It is a very frustrating experience for the patient and his family, as it often is for the ED staff as well.

The admission process may also require initial authorization by the insurance company or payor. The ED staff will call the insurance company and provide the clinical justification for a hospitalization. From a practical standpoint, the insurance company is looking for evidence of dangerousness or an inability to care for oneself because of a mental illness. Their goal is to authorize the least expensive level of care that is consistent with the patient's safety. If the admission is denied by the payor, either a lower level of care is authorized (such as a partial hospitalization program) or the ED staff must appeal the denial. This is done by phone, and another clinician for the insurance company reviews the information. This appeal is often unsuccessful, which may lead to a doc-to-doc review, where a psychiatrist contracted by the insurance company discusses the case with the ED physician or the consulting psychiatrist in the ED to settle on a plan. There is an art to this type of negotiation, but it is often quite frustrating for the physician in the Emergency Department when a remote insurance company physician, who has never laid eyes on the patient, tells the doctor who has actually examined the patient what constitutes appropriate treatment. Usually, the right decisions are made (meaning the insurance company doctor usually authorizes the admission that the ED physician requests), but these negotiations take a lot of time and divert resources away from patient care. Another patient in the ED may be waiting for an evaluation, but the clinicians may be busy negotiating with hospitals for beds and with insurance companies for authorizations. Rarely, a doctor must appeal a denial to the state insurance commissioner's office for a final determination, though an angry phone call from a family member to the insurance company's medical director can be surprisingly effective.

There is a great deal of subjectivity to this interhospital communication when reviewing a patient for possible transfer. Like it or not, the personalities of the ED staff and the unit staff come into play and will sometimes affect these decisions. The goal of the unit staff members is to get a realistic assessment of the patient's needs and determine if they can manage those needs; they don't want to accept a new patient only to learn he needs more care than they can offer. The goal of the ED staff is to find a place that will accept the patient. If a patient is accepted but the patient's symptoms on arrival turn out to be more acute than the staff were told (e.g., if the patient is aggressive, or requires increased supervision or a quiet room), then the nurses on that unit are less likely to believe those same ED staff members the next time they call to offer a patient for transfer. Memories of past perceived deceptions like this can last a long time.

Mitchell waited with his mother for many hours. She wanted him to take off his coat, but he insisted he was fine and fell asleep for a while on an uncomfortable chair. She went to the cafeteria and brought him back a sandwich and a Coke because he didn't trust the food that his nurse had brought him. Other patients came and went from the psychiatry area of the ED. One woman with two-tone hair paced and mumbled. Another gentleman sat quietly staring at his feet. Everyone was impatient.

Finally, they were told that Mitchell had been cleared for admission to a nearby psychiatric hospital. He needed to sign papers saying he was going voluntarily; then he would be transported to the hospital by ambulance. His mother could meet him there, where the admission office would have more paperwork for him.

"What if I don't want to stay?" Mitchell asked.

"You've signed in voluntarily, so you can sign yourself out." Uninformed or hurried ED staff will sometimes make this promise without explaining the exceptions. In our state, a patient must provide a 72-hour notice to leave before the team feels he is ready. This gives the hospital up to three days to be certain that the patient presents a low risk of danger to himself or others. Prior to the end of 72 hours, if there is the risk of danger and the patient still wants to leave, a hospital can then certify the patient, and the mechanism switches to the involuntary commitment process that happened with Josh in chapter 2. If he does not meet certification criteria, the treatment team has the option to release a patient sooner than 72 hours. This was all explained to Mitchell, and he signed the voluntary admission agreement and went to the new hospital.

Many patients enter an inpatient psychiatric unit for the first time having no idea what to expect. Once accepted, the patient is sent via ambulance to the receiving hospital. Family often want to transfer the patient themselves rather than by ambulance, but this is generally not permitted because the transferring hospital remains accountable for ensuring that the patient is safely transferred to the receiving facility. When the patient arrives, the receiving hospital reviews the paperwork for completeness and gives the patient a tour of the unit, followed by the nursing assessment. Typically, during the first 24 hours, the patient is also assessed by a social worker and a psychiatrist, and some units also have psychologists and occupational therapists.

Other professionals on the hospital unit may include art and music therapists and substance abuse counselors. A physical exam is performed, sometimes by the psychiatric physician but usually by an internist, nurse practitioner, or physician's assistant. Each discipline provides a different domain of expertise to assess the patient's needs and to provide recommendations for addressing these needs. These phases run parallel to each other, because discharge planning begins at admission.

What are the goals for a psychiatric hospitalization? The main goals are to identify the problems, to decide on interventions, and to initiate these treatments. These goals are reflected in the three main phases of inpatient hospitalization, which are assessment, treatment, and discharge planning.

The assessment phase includes interviewing the patient and relevant collateral sources of information (the family, co-workers, friends, therapists, other physicians) about current and past symptoms and treatments, reviewing records, and determining the most likely diagnosis or diagnoses. Other problems are identified, such as housing and financial difficulties, occupational factors, relationship problems, and barriers to accessing health care, such as being uninsured or having transportation problems. Additional laboratory data are collected, if indicated, to look for evidence of endocrine disorders, kidney or liver disease, blood or vitamin problems, and drug or alcohol issues. Sometimes, brain imaging studies, such as MRIs or CT scans, or electrical recordings of the brain (EEGs) are obtained to better assess brain function. Psychological and neuropsychological tests are sometimes used to help characterize problem areas. All this information is put together and analyzed so that a successful treatment plan can be developed.

The treatment plan is typically developed using a team approach, and each member (including the patient) suggests interventions to address the identified problems. The amount of participation by the patient in this plan varies from place to place; greater involvement usually leads to more treatment satisfaction.

Medication changes are often the key treatment plan item that an insurance company is interested in. Medication suggestions are reviewed, based on diagnosis, symptoms, medical history, family history, prior medication experiences, and patient preferences regarding desirable and undesirable side effects. A thoughtful psychiatrist will take the time to explore the patient's preferences and concerns and to help him make a carefully considered decision about whether to start a medication and which one to select.

Mitchell was very quiet on the unit, and he didn't want to participate in groups or occupational therapy. He didn't even want to take off his coat for the first couple of days, and he refused to bathe, even when the nurse gently informed him that he smelled. He watched a little TV, but he seemed to be quite suspicious. Jackie, his nurse, brought him some medicine, but he did not want to take it.

"How's that going to help?" Mitchell asked Jackie.

"It might help the voices go away. It could make you feel more comfortable and help you to worry less."

"I need to be alert," Mitchell said. To Mitchell, there were many reasons not to take the medicine. Anyone in such circumstances should be worried, as he was being watched by the authorities!

The psychiatrist, Dr. Susan Santos, met with Mitchell every day. He was getting no better, and he refused to even try medications. The health insurance company was asking her to discharge him: why be in the hospital if he wasn't going to take medications? She continued to talk to Mitchell about his concerns about taking medicines, and he did reluctantly agree to at least try.

Education is another treatment intervention that is important in the inpatient setting. Patients are taught about their particular illness; they identify behaviors and events that might trigger a relapse; and they learn coping strategies that help to improve symptoms and prevent relapse.

Education about medications is also important, particularly about the amount of time it takes for them to work, the possible side effects, and how to manage them. Education is very much a participatory experience, unlike many other medical settings in which the patient just does as he is told.

Family involvement is also important in most situations. Having at least one family meeting, either in person or by teleconference, is common on an inpatient treatment plan. This permits family members to express their observations and concerns and helps the clinicians understand the family dynamics that may impede or promote a patient's progress.

Formal talk therapy, or psychotherapy, is used less frequently in inpatient settings than it used to be. The average stay now lasts four to eight days, which does not provide much time for psychotherapy to be useful, though a number of short-term forms of psychotherapy are useful, such as supportive and cognitive-behavioral therapies. More common is group therapy, which is the mainstay of inpatient psychiatric treatment. Most units will have four to six group sessions per day, with different goals for each of the groups. Some examples of group therapy include stress management and problem-solving sessions.

Milieu therapy is another component of inpatient treatment. This term implies that the hospital unit is a therapeutic community and that most aspects of the inpatient experience are designed to have some therapeutic benefit. The word *milieu* refers to the environment. Patients eat meals in a common day area, play games that emphasize interpersonal communication, and even watch movies at night with themes they might discuss afterward. Clinical staff members observe patterns of interaction among the patients, and this helps them gauge the patients' ability to function outside the hospital. If a patient refuses to leave his bedroom and doesn't interact with others, it can be challenging to determine how prepared he is to go back to the community.

A nurse stood outside Mitchell's door with a towel.

"You need to take a shower, Mitchell," she said. She'd been suggesting this for some time, but now she was insisting. Mitchell smelled awful, and other patients were complaining. Some staff members didn't want to work with him because his odor was so offensive. Mitchell still didn't want to shower, and he was angry that people were insisting. Until now, he'd said little and had walked away when they'd told him to bathe.

"Get out of my face!" Mitchell yelled. He started pacing, and then he got very close to the nurse. She stepped back.

"Calm down, Mitchell, and go back in your room for now."

"Bitch! Bitch! Devil bitch! Six degrees of heaven and hell!" Mitchell yelled, and he moved faster, straight toward the nurse. Another patient yelled out while a different nurse hit an emergency buzzer on the wall. Mitchell grabbed the nurse's wrist and snatched the towel, all the while screaming obscenities. Soon patients gathered to watch, and security guards came running. Mitchell let go and the nurse stepped away, obviously shaken. A large male psychiatrist tried to talk to Mitchell, who kept screaming and would not calm down. When he stepped toward the psychiatrist with a raised fist, three security guards grabbed him, deftly restrained him, and escorted him into a seclusion room. He remained agitated and was given an injection of a sedating medication.

Sometimes a patient on an inpatient unit will become so agitated and upset that he will be asked to go to the quiet room, sometimes called the seclusion room. This is sometimes misunderstood to be a punishment, and indeed, the quiet room has no doubt been misused in that way. A quiet room is a place that is removed from the hubbub of the rest of the unit, where the patient can be away from the disruptive influence of others and can settle down, meditate, or rest. Patients are often encouraged to use the quiet room when they feel the need to take a break, as a form of self-regulation, particularly if there is a concern that they may become threatening or violent. When someone is really out of control and disruptive to the unit, he may be forced to enter the quiet room until he regains control. A distinction is made between an open door and a closed door quiet room. The door is closed and locked when a patient is so out of control that he is disruptive or a danger to others and refuses to remain in the open door quiet room. In extreme situations, he may be placed in restraints, with three or four limbs tied down to restrict his movement. Restraint is only performed when the patient is imminently dangerous to himself or others and no other intervention has been helpful. This is sometimes another one of those difficult decisions we have to make to balance safety with freedom. In Mitchell's case, there were no other options because he was an imminent danger, first to the nurse, and then to everyone else around him.

Any time a patient is involuntarily restricted to a room, it is considered to be *seclusion*, and when a patient's body part, such as a limb or torso, is restricted from movement, it is considered to be *restraint*. Regulations and state laws limit the application of seclusion and restraint to very specific circumstances. Hospitals are required to track their use of restraint and seclusion, and these statistics are part of a hospital's *core measures*, which are reported to the Joint Commission, an agency that accredits hospitals. Hospitals work toward becoming totally restraint-free and seclusion-free by improving the ability of their staff to help patients de-escalate their agitated or aggressive behaviors. Staff can also work to help patients identify what specific interventions they prefer to use when their behavior begins to escalate.

In the past, restraint and seclusion were used as forms of "treatment" because there were no medications to treat mental illness. They were overused and used inappropriately. In the first part of the twentieth century, more humane methods for treatment of "the insane" were adopted, and in 1956, the Mental Health Bell was crafted from melted iron shackles removed from the asylums of the day. This bell remains the symbol of Mental Health America, one of the largest mental health advocacy organizations in the United States. The bell's inscription reads: "Cast from shackles which bound them, this bell shall ring out hope for the mentally ill and victory over mental illness."

Mitchell fell asleep in the seclusion room and stayed there for the night. A staff member sat outside, and once it was clear that Mitchell was no longer agitated, the door was left open. Food and water were brought, but Mitchell remained asleep. A nurse checked his vital signs.

When Mitchell woke up, he was much calmer. The injection they had used to sedate him was also an antipsychotic medication, and it helped him feel a bit better. The nurse handed him a pill with water, and for the first time, Mitchell willingly took the medication. He was asked if he felt he could be safe if he left the quiet room, and he agreed. The nurse suggested he might want to take a shower and join one of the groups, and Mitchell did this.

As Mitchell was going to group, he passed several patients sitting in the hall in wheelchairs. They were not going to group therapy, and they had not eaten breakfast. They were waiting for electroconvulsive therapy (ECT), more commonly known as shock treatments.

ECT is one of the most effective forms of treatment for severe major depression that we have in our toolkit. Mention ECT, however, and people may recall the image of actor Jack Nicholson getting ECT—without anesthesia—for being a troublemaker in the 1975 movie *One Flew Over the Cuckoo's Nest*.

ECT involves giving an electrical pulse to the brain, typically lasting about two seconds, which causes the brain to have a seizure. It's the seizure, not the electricity, that has the therapeutic effect. The most effective seizure will last twenty to thirty seconds, so the electrical pulse is adjusted to induce a seizure of this length. Short-acting anesthesia is used to render the patient unconscious, and paralyzing agents are used to prevent painful and harmful muscle contraction. The patient is typically unconscious for only five minutes or so and often will not have any memories of events immediately before the treatment. Memory loss may occur from several minutes to hours before or after the seizure, though much longer periods of amnesia may happen rarely. The usual course is six to twelve treatments, administered three times per week, so it takes two to four weeks for the complete course. The first few treatments are often started while the person is an inpatient and can be completed as an outpatient. The risks of treatment include headaches after the procedure, the risks of anesthesia, and problems with memory loss, which can be significant for some patients. Modern ECT is a safe and effective form of treatment for severe depression but is used only in severe or treatment-resistant cases of depression because of the expense, the stigma, and the risk of memory loss.

Mitchell never became very talkative in the hospital, and he never did much on his own initiative. He agreed to take medications and to participate in his treatment, though it was never clear whether he wanted this or whether it was the path of least resistance. His behavior gradually became more organized, and he said the voices were quieter. He seemed to worry less about a conspiracy against him, but he never felt that it hadn't been real. Shortly, the psychiatrist told him he could go home. His mother was not happy.

"Mitchell is finally getting treatment! Why are you discharging him now? He's getting better, but he's still hearing voices, and he has a long way to go until he's ready to function well in society. Can you see him looking for a job like this?" she asked the doctor.

"I agree," the psychiatrist said, "but he can get further treatment as an outpatient. He doesn't need to be in the hospital any longer."

"But what if he stops taking medicine or won't go to his appointments? How do you know what he needs? Why stop now? You're doing a great job, and he's getting better, and it's only been twelve days!"

"I know, and I agree that Mitchell would probably benefit from a longer hospitalization. But the insurance company won't pay for hospitalization any longer, which means that Mitchell would get saddled with the debt. They only pay for patients who are acutely ill and actively dangerous. Mitchell's problem is more chronic, and he appears safe to leave now."

Many insurance companies review the progress of an inpatient every couple of days. If it appears that no active treatment is being provided, for example, if there are no medication changes in several days, or if the patient has reached a maximum level of improvement, then they may stop paying for the care. This review is called a *continued stay authorization*, and is part of the *prospective review process*. If this authorization is denied for lack of medical necessity, then the patient may be discharged, if clinically appropriate, or be kept in the hospital while an appeal process is followed, which occurs if the treatment team believes the patient is not yet stable for discharge. This appeal process may not get resolved until long after a patient is discharged. When such a delay occurs, it becomes part of the *retrospective review process*; a copy of the entire chart is sent to the insurance company, which makes a determination based on its own continued stay criteria. These processes have an impact on decisions that are made about treatment.

After the patient is initially assessed, a set of problems identified, and a treatment plan initiated, the staff begins to formulate a discharge plan. Various concerns are taken into consideration in the discharge plan, such as where the person will live, who will provide aftercare treatment, and how the person will get medications. All these factors can have an impact on the length of stay in the hospital, but the most important factors are the patient's safety and the likelihood of imminent rehospitalization. Once the patient is no longer a risk to himself or to others, then discharge can be considered.

It is surprising what can be accomplished in a five-day hospital stay. This brief stay becomes a crisis intervention and stabilization tool more than a long-term treatment intervention. The treatment team helps cool down the situation, assesses what is wrong and what is needed, points the person in the right direction, and then helps her on her way. Outpatient follow-up is critical to ensuring that interventions started on the inpatient unit can be carried over into the outpatient realm.

Some people still come into the hospital requesting long-term hospitalization. This doesn't exist anymore, for the most part. In the 1950s, there were over 500,000 state psychiatric hospital beds in the United States, and there are now under 50,000. There will likely be fewer beds in the near future as states continue to cut their budgets. This was a result of the de-institutionalization movement, which was ignited by the development of effective medications for psychotic illnesses like schizophrenia. Since then, laws have required that people be treated in the least restrictive environment, meaning that if they can be treated in the community, then they must be discharged from the hospital.

As states have enjoyed the reductions in costs associated with fewer state hospital beds, they have steadily shut down these facilities. Many states have devoted all or part of the money that used to go toward inpatient treatment to the development and maintenance of outpatient community treatment, including therapeutic group homes and crisis beds. The remaining state psychiatric beds are largely for forensic patients who are committed there by the court, often as part of a pretrial assessment to determine their capacity to stand trial. In Maryland, more than two-thirds of our state hospital beds are now taken up by forensic patients. The remainder are filled mostly by patients with severe and persistent mental illnesses who cannot be managed in a community setting. The days when a patient could be quickly admitted to a state hospital are just about over.

Many believe this to be a good thing, because patients with mental illness, or any illness for that matter, should be treated as close to their home and family as possible. Being sent to a state hospital can be very stigmatizing. There is no reason general hospitals should not have psychiatric units, just as they have cardiac units, pediatric units, and OB units. Others believe this mainstreaming of mental illness treatment within the larger medical domain is a detriment to progressive psychiatric care. And some believe that a segment of ill patients benefit from long-term care; without state hospital beds, this option exists only for insanity acquittees and the financially well-off, who can afford treatment at the handful of long-term psychiatric hospitals that remain.

Many people are unaware of the financial stigma that psychiatric units have with administrators of general hospitals. Psychiatric beds are among the lowest reimbursed bed categories in hospital settings, often losing money. They are maintained by many hospitals to meet the needs of the community, and they provide a service to patients who might otherwise be boarding in the ED for days. Many hospitals, however, choose to forego the responsibility of providing inpatient psychiatric care and instead elect to have beds that bring in more dollars per square foot per day. Patients sometimes find it hard to think of the hospital as a business that must operate with a positive margin, but that is what it takes for hospitals to stay open. If a hospital lacks sufficient psychiatric beds, writing letters to the hospital and to community leaders may help to remind them of this community responsibility.

Discharge planning really starts at admission, when the social worker assesses the patient's ability to return to the preadmission living situation. With Mitchell, there was no question; he'd go home to live with his mom. Once the post-discharge housing situation is clarified, the aftercare treatment can be arranged, either with the patient's current providers or with new ones. These providers may include a psychiatrist or a therapist or both. Great effort is made to get these appointments arranged for soon after discharge, which increases the likelihood of a smooth transition of care. In fact, one of the core measures of quality selected by the Joint

Commission is the percentage of discharge plans that are documented to have been transmitted to aftercare providers. Unfortunately, the communication between inpatient and outpatient providers is often inadequate. Sometimes a patient shows up for an outpatient appointment and the doctor knows nothing about what happened during the hospitalization except what the patient tells him. Patients often don't remember the names of their medications, the doses they were prescribed, or the results of the testing that was done.

Mitchell's mother went with him to see a psychiatrist after he left the hospital. She brought the bottles of medication that he was taking, and she knew that Mitchell's blood work was all normal and that a brain scan had also been normal. While Mitchell said very little, his mother was able to tell the doctor that he was much better than he had been in the hospital. The doctor asked him to sign an authorization to release his information so that he could get records from the hospital.

"Just look in the computer," Mitchell said.

"The computer?" the new psychiatrist asked. He wondered if Mitchell was having delusions about technology!

"In the hospital, all the records are on the computer."

Mitchell wasn't delusional about this at all; the hospital kept an electronic record of all tests, medications, consults, and hospital stays. What was not obvious to Mitchell was that these records could be accessed only by people inside the hospital, and the new psychiatrist could not see them from the computer on his desk.

Poor communication is, of course, a problem that besets all health care in the United States. One way to improve communication is to share medical records and information. This has traditionally been done via phone call and mail. In the 1980s, fax machines became a quicker method to transmit medical information about a patient. You'd think that in 2011, with e-mail and the Internet, we'd have much more efficient and effective methods for sharing this information, but we are not quite there.

The practice of medicine has used paper records for centuries, and despite the availability of personal computers for the past thirty years, physicians and hospitals have been slow to adopt electronic health records (EHRs), which are also sometimes referred to as electronic medical records (EMRs).

Since the 1960s, there have been attempts to computerize patient records. The problem with paper records is that pertinent information may exist in one doctor's file that another doctor never knows about. Even within a provider's record, pertinent information may get lost. In addition, there has been an increasing trend toward fragmented health care relationships as patients have frequent health insurance changes. Physicians also change their health insurance network affiliations, move, change jobs, and alter their practice styles in ways that may not be conducive to long-term doctor-patient relationships.

President George W. Bush began an initiative that would create the National Health Information Network (NHIN), a system of secure data networks that pools a patient's health information together in some coherent manner, connecting numerous EHRs to improve the delivery of effective and efficient health care. The potential benefits of this health care information technology include improved care by facilitating communication between providers, reduced healthcare costs by improving efficiency and reducing repetitive tests, and increased medical knowledge by collecting aggregate data about diseases for research and education.

The potential risks of EHRs are frequently discussed as well, including threats to information security, unintended uses of the data that are collected, breaches of confidentiality, and loss of independent medical decision making by physicians who fear that computer algorithms will supplant our human ones.

Some electronic records stylize doctor notes with checkbox forms in place of narrative descriptions of symptoms and circumstance, deliberations about diagnostic reasoning, and thoughtful discussions of treatment options. In psychiatry, these checkbox formats drain our clinical work of its richness. Instead of being able to document that the patient "believed he was the president, so he hopped on a bus to Washington, camped out on Pennsylvania Avenue for three weeks, then climbed over the fence of the White House," the scenario may be reduced to one little box that says "delusional." We treat people through language and free communication. Current information systems tend to stifle the nuances. Better electronic systems allow for thoughtful narratives about patient care, particularly in psychiatry.

EHRs can influence treatment in other ways. Some systems have pop-up warnings about drug interactions. Although this is potentially helpful, if not life saving, its usefulness gets lost if the warnings include insignificant, minor, and very rare interactions, and if the quantity of the pop-ups is so great that significant warnings get lost in the muddle of alerts. The key to developing truly functional EHRs with excellent user interfaces is to include clinicians in the planning and development process.

Privacy and security are other areas of concern with EHRs, especially since health care providers and patients are expected to use and trust these products with their personal health information. Part of the national discussion includes the question of who owns a patient's personal health information (PHI). According to HIPAA, patients have a right to receive a copy of their records, electronically if they prefer. They may also control who has access to their information. But most patients who try to access their records, or to determine who has viewed them, face many barriers in getting this information. One of the solutions has been personal health records (PHRs), in which patients have more control over the data that gets placed in their record and more control over who gets to see it. Both Google Health and Microsoft HealthVault are products that allow people to place their own PHI online. Patients then control who has access to it. Patients can allow doctors, hospitals, and family to read all or parts of their medical record.

The problem with EHRs and PHRs is that they wind up being silos or slices of health data, and no single place exists where all available health information is tied together for any given patient. One of the patient-centered groups that has been pushing for an open standard for communicating health data is *SpeakFlower.org*, whose mission is to advocate for a common "language" so that patients, doctors, and facilities can talk and share health data in real time, when needed and as authorized. This would have been helpful to the psychiatrist who saw Mitchell after he left the hospital, and perhaps Mitchell envisioned such an efficient system when he assumed the psychiatrist could access inpatient information on the computer.

Another group is *healthdatarights.org*, which has proposed a Declaration of Health Data Rights stating that all patients:

- Have the right to their own health data
- Have the right to know the source of each health data element
- Have the right to take possession of a complete copy of their individual health data, without delay, at minimal or no cost; if data exist in computable form, they must be made available in that form
- Have the right to share their health data with others as they see fit

Over 1,400 organizations and individuals have endorsed this declaration, though it has yet to be adopted by the Health Information Technology Policy Committee that sets national policies for health information technology.

The ONC, or Office of the National Coordinator for Health Information Technology (also called ONCHIT), is the federal agency that is developing national standards to address these issues. The 2009 stimulus bill included the HITECH Act. This act established $19 billion in stimulus funds designed to encourage hospitals and health care providers to adopt certified EHRs and use them in a meaningful way. The actual definition of "meaningful use" was finalized in 2010. The Certification Commission for Health Information Technology (CCHIT) is the main group that certifies EHRs, and in July 2010, they began certifying behavioral health EHRs. This certification has privacy and security requirements that improve the safety and accuracy of behavioral health care notes and information.

Patients who are receiving behavioral health care may be interested in knowing how their personal information is protected. A truly engaged patient (often called an e-patient) might ask his provider if she is using an EHR, and if the EHR is certified. Other questions might include whether the data are stored "in the cloud," who else has access to the data, and if an audit trail of access is maintained. *The cloud* refers to a distributed model of data storage where files are maintained on file servers that are connected to the Internet and available from any other computer using the proper authorization procedures. A patient may also ask to receive electronic copies of his records to import into his PHR of choice, though at this time, few clinicians are prepared to do this, and many may not even understand these concepts.

Access to these larger amounts of personal health information will no doubt transform the practice of medicine and the way patients manage their health information. The resulting changes to the practice of psychiatry are expected to be dramatic and will, we hope, result in an improvement in the health of people with chronic mental illnesses while further reducing the stigma of these diseases.

Will the benefits of a national health information system outweigh the risks? Better yet, will doctors and patients be able to use it without wanting to throw the computer out the window? Only time will tell. Health information technology brings much promise to the future of health care, but we must learn how to use this technology well while providing safe health care. It's like operating on a malfunctioning heart while it is still beating; it must be accomplished carefully because the consequences of mistakes can be quite serious. At this time, many patients worry about the potential for wrong information to be recorded and transmitted. Others express concerns about who exactly can see their psychiatric information. Some patients worry that electronic records will allow their dermatologist to know the details of their psychiatric histories when they'd like the option of keeping that information to themselves. Worse, others worry that their colleagues, neighbors, and employers might access private information through computer systems, and the EHRs in use vary greatly in accessibility. These can be very real concerns for patients. Most systems track users and the information they access. Physicians have even been fired from their jobs for accessing information about people who are not their patients. Some patients want their privacy for inappropriate reasons—for example, a patient may be obtaining pain medications from several physicians to maintain an addiction, and these doctors might not be willing to prescribe if an EHR alerted them to this. The trust in these systems would increase if patients could access their EHR at any time and review the audit trail of who accessed which information for what purpose. Finally, people worry that medical information may be accessed by insurance companies, who might then deny patients either health or life insurance. Employers, camps, schools, and licensing boards already require people to divulge medical and psychiatric information. Might they require applicants to allow access to their EHRs? This seems unlikely, but it is not unreasonable for patients and physicians to worry about how their information will be used, and these issues are still being considered as the technology develops.

Mitchell's mother didn't feel he was really ready to go home. He was still hearing voices, but he was beginning to recognize them as hallucinations. He still worried a lot, and he didn't do much at home. He hadn't been to school in a long time, and his mother hoped he might think about getting a job, but he was still struggling.

The psychiatrist did not think Mitchell was sick enough to be in the hospital, but he did agree that Mitchell needed a more intensive level of treatment than he could offer in his office. He referred Mitchell to a psychiatric day hospital for ongoing care.

Partial hospitalization programs (PHP), also called day hospitals, are often located at a hospital center and provide intensive outpatient treatment for a good portion of the day. PHPs are intended to provide much of the benefit of an inpatient treatment but in an outpatient setting. Patients usually attend PHPs for three to five days a week, usually for six hours daily. Most of that time is spent in group therapy and education sessions, with time also spent in individual therapy, medication management, and family therapy.

PHPs are used both as step-down units after an inpatient hospitalization and as intensive treatment programs as an alternative to hospitalization. These are good treatment programs for people who need more care but who want to go home at night. The cost of a PHP course of treatment, often lasting two to three weeks, can be a quarter to a third of the cost of a five- to seven-day inpatient hospitalization. Some PHPs specialize in the populations they treat, such as adolescents or the elderly. There are day hospitals for substance abuse, eating disorders, and mood disorders. Others take a more general approach.

Some hospitals also have outpatient clinics where people receive much less intensive treatment than at PHPs. Hospital-based outpatient clinics tend to be more expensive to run than private outpatient clinics, which don't carry the associated expenses of a large hospital. Whether or not a hospital has an outpatient clinic is often related to how the hospital is funded for such treatments and whether the hospital has the available space for such a facility. Teaching hospitals often establish them as a training ground for residents or as a recruitment pool for research studies.

Mitchell felt much better emotionally. He took several medications, and he came to realize that the medicines helped him.

One day he had a high fever, his stomach hurt terribly, and he vomited. Hours went by, and he got worse. He called his primary care doctor, then went to the emergency room. By the time he got to surgery, his appendix had ruptured. Mitchell spent several days in the hospital getting intravenous antibiotics and healing from his operation. He told the surgeon the names of the medicines he took, and the surgeon was unfamiliar with them. Even though Mitchell's behavior was fine and he seemed to be doing well, the surgeon called for a psychiatry consult.

The final type of hospital-based psychiatric activity we will discuss is the consultation service to medical and surgical floors. This has historically been referred to as *consultation-liaison (C-L) psychiatry*, but the term *psychosomatic medicine* has been used more recently. These consultations are done by psychiatrists who have experience providing psychiatric consultations to other physicians in a hospital setting, mostly for patients who are admitted to the medical or surgical unit in the hospital.

Physicians admitting a patient to their service for a medical condition, for example pneumonia, might request a consultation from a C-L psychiatrist if the patient starts to hallucinate, acts very confused, or becomes very depressed. The consultation-liaison psychiatrist may get called to see someone who has taken an overdose, shot himself in a suicide attempt, or made a statement that he wishes he were dead. Other reasons for consult requests include management of alcohol or drug withdrawal, assessment for dementia, or evaluation of someone's current medications. Hospital psychiatrists are also involved in evaluating someone's ability to make rational decisions, just as we discussed in chapter 7, when Eddie's mother, Susan, was dying of AIDS and wanted to leave the hospital. Sometimes a consult is called because the treating doctor cannot find a medical explanation for the patient's symptoms and begins to wonder whether the problems might have a psychiatric cause, especially if the patient has a history of psychiatric problems or is on a psychotropic medication. Unfortunately, some physicians let this history cloud their judgment and may dismiss or perform inadequate diagnostic workups of physical symptoms in patients with psychiatric disorders.

Evaluating a patient who is on the medical service requires a different approach from the psychiatrist. The first thing the psychiatrist must do is put the patient at ease and establish a rapport. Many patients' first reaction is to assume that their doctor thinks they are crazy.

We usually tell these medical patients that most of the patients we see are not crazy but are having problems with coping or with their brain reacting to their medical problem or to a medication, and that our job is to figure out what is wrong and how to fix it. We've had many people refuse to talk to us. "I don't need a psychiatrist," they say. We might not immediately start out with "Hi, I'm a psychiatrist." Instead we tell them why we were asked to see them and find out what problems they are experiencing. One of the most enjoyable activities in psychiatry is that initial visit when one first meets a person and engages with them toward understanding what the problems are and how to address them.

Otherwise, the approach on the medical unit is like that on the psychiatric unit: assessment, treatment, and discharge; however, these steps must be accomplished in very little time. Much of the assessment occurs by reviewing the record, talking with the attending physician and family, and taking a good history from the patient. The diagnosis and treatment recommendations are then laid out, followed by any aftercare advice. Helping the patient get connected to community resources is also a common task of the C-L psychiatrist. In Mitchell's case, the psychiatrist reviewed his history and medications, called his outpatient psychiatrist, and assured the surgeon that he would be available if any psychiatric concerns came up. Mitchell did need to remain on his medications while he was in the hospital, but for several days he couldn't eat, and the psychiatrist asked that he be given a couple of doses by injection, just to be sure he remained well, and Mitchell was fine with this.

On the business side of C-L psychiatry, hospitals usually have to subsidize the psychiatrist since it is common for C-L psychiatrists to collect less than fifteen to twenty cents on the dollar due to complex insurance rules about whether they will pay for psychiatric diagnostic codes. Hospitals benefit from these consultations by having behavior problems addressed, medicolegal issues well managed, and length of stay improved. The hospital may also get reimbursed better for some patients because a psychiatric illness may increase the severity of the patient's problem, and hospitals are reimbursed according to patients' diagnostic-related groups (DRGs). This can amount to an average of three hundred to four hundred dollars in additional revenue per psychiatric consultation, though this goes to the hospital not the physician.

Mitchell got better in a sense. Medications controlled his symptoms, he was much easier to live with, and he helped out at home. He enjoyed family events, and he enrolled in a program to help people with chronic mental illnesses get jobs. He never fully went back to being the person he had been before he got sick, and he never had a lot of initiative or motivation to try new things on his own. Every few years, he tried to go off his medications, just to see if he could, and twice he ended up in the hospital. Mitchell's schizophrenia was a devastating illness for him and his mother, but they learned to live with it, and he got excellent care.

Chapter 10

Sharon:
The Business of Psychiatry

SHARON BUCHANAN'S DOCTOR was very worried about her weight loss.
He thought she might have cancer, and he was about to order a number
of tests when she confessed that she was actively dieting and exercising
for hours a day. She wanted to be even thinner and was terrified of becoming fat.

"But you look like a skeleton, and 110 is just not a healthy weight for a
woman of 5 feet 6 inches. You have anorexia," he said. He gave her the
name of a well-respected psychiatrist and told her she had to go.

Sharon called, but the psychiatrist was not in her insurance network;
in fact, he wasn't in any of the insurance networks. She called her doctor
back and asked for another name.

"I want you to see the psychiatrist I suggested. He's the best doctor in
town, and he specializes in eating disorders. I don't want you to see just
any psychiatrist."

So far, we've talked about psychiatry as a medical specialty, and we've
examined issues mostly from a patient's perspective. In this chapter, we
talk about psychiatric practice from the doctor's perspective, specifically
the business aspects of being a psychiatrist. As doctors, we don't usually
discuss these features of our work with those outside the field, but we
think it's necessary to show what's "behind the curtain" so that others
really understand how psychiatrists come to practice as they do.

The financial aspects of psychiatric care can be an uncomfortable
topic for everyone. Patients who are ill and suffering often aren't up to

the task of negotiating payment for services, and usually payment is necessary to get treatment. Psychiatrists know that treatment is expensive and that patients sometimes must balance the cost of care against the price of other necessities; however, we also know that psychiatric conditions have many hidden costs: the immeasurable cost of psychic suffering and the very real cost of lost income due to disability or unmet occupational potential. We also have our own bills and financial obligations. Because people share such intimate details of their lives with their psychiatrists, and because treatment can last for years, patients often begin to relate to their therapists as confidantes and friends, and the payment of fees is an intrusive reminder that the relationship is a business endeavor that includes something more than the psychiatrist's concern for the patient's well-being.

Increasingly, medical care is not simply an exchange of a service for a fee but is a complicated interaction between insurance companies, their managed care agencies, and the psychiatrist. These agencies may dictate what types of problems are eligible for reimbursement and under what conditions. And it's not just the private practice clinician who has to be aware of financial matters: they affect hospitals, clinics, correctional facilities, day programs, and emergency departments as well.

Patients discover the financial aspect of mental health care when they make the first call for treatment. Like Sharon, they may learn that the psychiatrist they'd like to see does not participate in their insurance network and then need to figure out if they have out-of-network benefits to help cover the cost, if they will pay for treatment out-of-pocket, or if they will search for another doctor. A patient who calls a clinic may discover that the clinic does not accept private insurance at all, or only accepts patients who live in a very specific geographic area. And in both private and public settings, there may be a long wait until an appointment is available. Even in the emergency room, questions are raised about insurance, finances, and who is responsible for the bill.

Psychiatrists—perhaps more than most other medical specialists—may not participate in health insurance plans. Even when the insurance company has a large list of in-network psychiatrists, the list may not be up to date or may contain doctors who aren't accepting new patients, doctors who limit their practices to certain conditions, or even doctors who are retired or dead. It may take several phone calls before a patient finds a participating psychiatrist who is taking new patients and who has the expertise that particular patient needs.

Why do doctors participate in insurance networks? Psychiatrists who are in-network may live in regions where there is a shortage of doctors and feel that insurance participation is the socially responsible thing to do so that people in their area have access to care. Others find that some insurers are easy to work with and do not feel overly burdened by their paperwork requirements. Finally, some psychiatrists do not get enough referrals to fill their practice unless they accept insurance. Financially, it may make sense to be an in-network psychiatrist if the doctor's practice has many patients who are seen only for brief medication management visits and are referred to other mental health professionals for psychotherapy. Participation may also make sense if the doctor divides his practice between medication management and psychotherapy.

Insurance companies reimburse at a higher hourly rate for several brief visits than for a single fifty-minute appointment, perhaps because they are eager to encourage their policyholders to seek psychotherapy with less expensive clinicians. A visit for medication management has no time restrictions on it as far as the insurance company is concerned. If a psychiatrist can see three or four patients in an hour, he can make a good income even with the constraints that insurance participation entails. An example might help to make this less confusing. To do this, we need to plug in some hypothetical fees, and we've chosen numbers that approximate the Medicare fees for our state. These fees depend on many things, including what type of facility the psychiatrist practices in and whether he participates with Medicare or not, and they are often well below the usual fees charged in private practice. We are just using these numbers to give an example.

A psychiatrist who sees a patient for a fifty-minute psychotherapy session with medication management may be reimbursed just under $105 a session. If the same psychiatrist sees a patient for twenty-five minutes for psychotherapy with medication management, the fee is just under $75, so the doctor's hourly rate is then around $150. For medication management without psychotherapy, the fee is approximately $55, so a psychiatrist who sees four patients in an hour will earn $220 an hour, or more than twice the rate of a doctor who sees only one patient for psychotherapy. Psychiatrists who do not accept insurance will also make more money by seeing more patients for less time, and many psychiatrists mix up their case loads to include some psychotherapy patients and some medication-only patients.

Is this bad? As we've said in earlier chapters, split therapy may not be the right kind of treatment for everyone, but many people who see psychiatrists for brief medication management appointments have improved lives and well-controlled illnesses. It's not the optimal treatment for every patient or every condition.

Sharon scheduled an appointment and called her insurance company. She had out-of-network benefits, so even though she would have to pay the doctor for the appointments, she could submit the bills for reimbursement.

"So, I'll get 80 percent back?" Sharon asked.

"There's a deductible," the secretary said, "and the managed care company needs to decide if your care is medically necessary, which they usually do, and then you can submit the bills, and they will send you 80 percent of their usual and customary fee."

"Is that the fee the doctor charges?" Sharon wanted to know.

"Not necessarily."

"So how much will an appointment cost me?"

"We can't say that in advance. You'll need to get preauthorized, and then you can submit the bills, and when you get a check, you'll know how much was covered. Please be aware that determination of medical necessity is not a guarantee of payment."

Sharon went to the appointment and paid for the professional fee by check but had no idea how much she'd get back from her insurance company.

Why don't all psychiatrists accept insurance? In short, because insurance companies often pay lower rates than psychiatrists want to charge, and because getting paid by an insurance company is a complicated and cumbersome process—so cumbersome that the reimbursement does not always make up for the time and expense of obtaining payment.

If a psychiatrist participates with an insurance network, that is, if he *accepts assignment*, then he agrees to practice according to the terms of the insurance company. He agrees to accept the fee that is set by the insurance company, which is called the usual and customary rate (UCR). The UCR is different for every insurance network. Insurance company UCRs are often lower than the fees that nonparticipating doctors set and may be much lower than the community's actual usual and customary standard for a service.

Furthermore, insurance policies issued by the same company may have different payment rates. For some insurance plans, there is a set co-pay, while for others, there may be a more complicated formula. For example, an insurance company may pay 80 percent for the first five visits and 70 percent for the next five visits and 60 percent for all the visits after that, and it may pay the percentage of its UCR, not a percentage of the doctor's regular fee. Sometimes patients are covered for only a certain number of visits, and part of the insurance agreement may be that the psychiatrist cannot bill the patient if care is required beyond what is covered.

For each patient, someone must call to verify the insurance, find out what the preauthorization involves, and determine the co-pays and yearly deductible. This work often involves lengthy phone calls, long periods on hold, and confusing telephone prompting menus. Some patients have two insurance policies, and then the work must be done with both the primary and the secondary insurance. For a psychiatrist who does psychotherapy and sees eight patients a day at an insurance company's discounted fee, the uncompensated time spent on paperwork and phone calls makes an insurance-based practice economically unfeasible.

To work as an in-network provider for insurance companies, most psychiatrists find they need to have a secretary, which is an overhead expense that an out-of-network doctor may not want or need. The office needs to be large enough to accommodate secretarial space, and the doctor's ability to earn an income is only as good as his secretary's skill at negotiating the insurance system to make sure that payment is collected. Many doctors use billing agencies instead, and these agencies are typically paid 7 percent of the doctors' collections. In either case, the money that is lost to administrative burdens is considerable.

Insurance participation with a given company is an all-or-nothing proposition. A psychiatrist can't accept insurance from one patient and request full payment from another patient with the same insurance, even if the patient is very wealthy or offers to pay for more intensive services. Sometimes, doctors have great trouble collecting fees from insurance companies, and patients may not always know if their doctor is getting paid for services rendered. In fact, the reimbursement process can be so confusing that even the doctor may not know if he is being compensated for his work.

Sometimes insurance companies find reasons to deny reimbursement after treatment is rendered. It is often difficult to collect fees from patients who were not expecting to pay, and participating psychiatrists may find they do work without pay. By not accepting assignment, the doctor has greater control over his fees, collections, and paperwork burden, and he may have lower overhead expenses.

If the patient sees an out-of-network doctor, then the patient bears the burden of negotiating the reimbursement process. The doctor requires payment from the patient in full, and the patient must request reimbursement directly from her insurance company for out-of-network care. This means that access to out-of-network psychiatric care is limited to those who have both the resources to pay for services up front and the organizational skills to call their managed care company for preauthorization and to submit the statements for reimbursement. Life is easier for the doctor, but it becomes more difficult for the patient. Clearly, something is broken with such a complicated and time-consuming system.

Going to a psychiatrist who is not on any insurance panel is not a guarantee of better care; however, Sharon's primary care doctor felt strongly that the care she'd get from this particular psychiatrist was better than what she'd get from someone else. He subtly implied that this psychiatrist was worth paying for. Insurance participation is much more about economic forces than it is about better or worse care, and in-network or out-of-network, patients may find clinicians who are helpful, knowledgeable, and comforting. When a patient is not satisfied with her treatment, however, she may want to seek a consultation, even if it means using out-of-network benefits or paying out-of-pocket. This may eliminate the intrusion of insurance companies and managed care organizations on treatment for difficult-to-treat conditions.

The Mental Health Parity and Addiction Equity Act of 2008 (also known as the Wellstone-Domenici Act), whose regulations went into effect in 2010, finally established rules that no longer permit insurance discrimination against mental health and substance abuse (MH/SA) disorders. Insurance plans offered by employers (except for small employers) must provide the same level of benefit for MH/SA disorders as they do for medical and surgical disorders. This means that insurance carriers can no longer establish separate quantitative (e.g., 20 visits per year; 50% co-pay for psychotherapy) or nonquantitative (e.g., time-consuming pre-authorization procedures; not covering residential psychiatric rehab but covering residential physical rehab) treatment limits. This applies to both in-network and out-of-network benefits. Until now, many insurance companies, even Medicare, were able to reimburse, say, 50 percent for mental health but 80 percent for physical health. Policing the timely implementation of these regulations will be a challenge. As insurance carriers adapt to these new rules, patients and providers will need to speak up and alert the proper regulating agencies when they see evidence of continued discrimination.

When we talk about the hassles of collection companies, we may sound unsympathetic to our patients' struggle with these same issues, as though we are whining about our paychecks. Most physicians still have comfortable lifestyles, though as with anyone, that can be defined by each person's standards. Many doctors feel that given the extensive years of training, the long hours of study, and the considerable cost it takes to become a physician, there is an expectation of a good lifestyle in exchange. Young doctors today sometimes graduate from medical school with hundreds of thousands of dollars in educational debt, and the stereotype of the rich doctor often does not hold up, or if it does, the wealth is a product of many years of hard work.

Sharon made the appointment with the psychiatrist, but the day came, and she forgot to go. The office called her, and she was embarrassed. "I completely forgot! My tennis partner got sick, and the game was rescheduled with another player who could only come at 11, and the appointment completely slipped my mind. I am so sorry! Can I reschedule for tomorrow?" Sharon asked. The secretary told her the doctor would be able to see her in two weeks and that there would be a fee for the missed appointment.

"That's ridiculous. I didn't even meet him! What a rip off."

"Yes, but the doctor held the time for you, and other patients who requested the appointment were told it was not available. He can't really run a practice if he doesn't charge people who forget to come."

"I'll think about it," Sharon said. She was not happy.

In addition to policies about payment procedures, psychiatrists often have policies that cover the issue of missed appointments. In a private psychotherapy practice, psychiatrists often run on time and don't double book, as internists or other doctors may do. Patients know that the time is theirs, and appointments must be canceled in advance. Late cancellations or unkept appointments are billed either in full or at a reduced cancellation rate. Some psychiatrists bill for all missed appointments; others make exceptions for illness and weather events.

From a psychiatrist's point of view, it can be very uncomfortable to charge for missed sessions when no service was rendered and there are valid reasons for missing appointments. Every patient has her own priority on keeping psychiatric appointments. While some patients never miss them, others cancel because of conflicting obligations or even simple inconveniences. It's also not uncommon for some patients to repeatedly forget appointments. While many doctors are willing to forgo their fee in the case of true emergencies, it is not feasible for most private practice doctors to run a business if they don't hold to some standard about charging for missed appointments. For a given doctor, this may depend on how big an issue it becomes in his practice. A psychiatrist who rarely has no-shows or late cancellations may be willing to dismiss these fees, but one who has this happen several times a week, or repeatedly with the same patients, may feel it necessary to charge for all missed appointments. When there is a financial disincentive for missing appointments, people are more careful about keeping them, and care is provided more consistently.

In public clinics, revenue comes from public payers, such as Medicare, Medicaid, and state funding to support care for the uninsured. In these settings, fees cannot be charged for missed appointments, and approximately 30 percent of appointments are not kept.

The issue of a no-show policy can be uncomfortable for both the patient and the doctor. Patients may resent being charged for a service they didn't receive and may quietly (or not so quietly!) resent their doctor, either for the financial loss or for the inconvenience of being held to the appointment. The psychiatrist may also begin to harbor some resentment toward patients who do not value the service and are not respectful of the time that is being set aside for them. Even if the doctor receives payment for the missed time, a no-show leaves him in a state of uncertainty, wondering if the patient is stuck in traffic, will be arriving soon, or is simply not coming. At any rate, these events can trigger unpleasant or uncharitable feelings for both the doctor and the patient, and either party may feel uncomfortable discussing them.

When someone misses sessions repeatedly, the issue can be used as a focus of treatment, and sometimes this is helpful. Other people who repeatedly miss appointments, however, grow comfortable with their irresponsibility as a way of life, or are unable to explore their motives beyond the superficial level of "I forgot." They may focus on blaming the external forces that prevent them from keeping appointments to receive treatment, and no good comes from missed appointments.

Sharon finally saw the doctor. He did a full psychiatric evaluation and also weighed her and took her blood pressure and pulse. They met several times, and then the psychiatrist suggested Sharon start a medication—not for anorexia, but for mood swings. The doctor told her the risks of the medication.

"You'll need to sign this form," he said, "and you'll have to get some labs done."

"Why do I need to sign a form to take a medication?" asked Sharon. "Is it that dangerous?"

"My malpractice agency thinks it is," he said. "They require that I get informed consent for certain classes of medication."

In addition to revenue concerns, expenses are also an issue for psychiatric practices. Psychiatrists in most states must purchase malpractice insurance, and concerns about the potential for litigation colors the way doctors practice. Increasingly, malpractice insurers and regulatory agencies dictate what the standards of care must be, and these standards are not necessarily the result of evidence-based research. Certainly, some of these mandates came about because poor care was being given, and they have fixed problems or helped to establish reasonable standards of care, but others have less to do with quality of care than with protection from liability. For example, some mental health systems require that the patient sign an informed consent document every time the dose of a medication is changed. Other systems require only an initial signed consent when a medication is prescribed for the first time. Some are less formal about informed consent and require only that a risk-benefit discussion be recorded in the progress note. Although informed consent is important, and we believe that patients should be educated about how their medications might help or harm them, requiring patients to sign forms does little to improve care while adding to the paperwork burden and creating an atmosphere of mistrust.

Signing a consent form for medications is only one example of something a psychiatrist might do to limit liability. Psychiatrists worry about other issues regarding standards of care to prevent successful lawsuits, and some of these are met with opposition by patients.

A psychiatrist may insist that a patient who is doing well must come to appointments with a certain frequency to get refills of medication, and this may represent a burden to a busy person who is not having symptoms and feels it should be adequate to tell the doctor on the phone that she is feeling well. The psychiatrist may believe the patient but may worry that if something should go wrong, he could be faulted for not having seen the patient in person in a long time.

Many medications are associated with adverse reactions that can be caught early with laboratory monitoring. Such reactions may be uncommon, but treatment standards still require that regular blood testing be done on patients who are taking certain medications. While these tests are done for a patient's protection, many people resist getting blood work done, and this can cause friction in the relationship between a psychiatrist and a patient. At times, it may become necessary for a psychiatrist to refuse to prescribe medications that have been very helpful if a patient will not get the necessary lab work, and every aspect of this gets troublesome. The doctor worries that the patient will relapse without the medication, but he also worries that he will be held responsible if a patient has a bad reaction to the medication, especially if the reaction could have been prevented by monitoring blood work.

How much a given doctor's practice is influenced by anxieties about potential litigation depends on various factors. Institutions such as hospitals, clinics, and correctional facilities may dictate fairly precise standards of care and documentation. Malpractice insurers may require doctors to get written informed consent for certain classes of medication or refuse to cover psychiatrists who offer unconventional treatments. Certainly a doctor who has already been sued will become very cautious, and unfortunately such experiences may lead psychiatrists to view their patients as potential adversaries. Finally, psychiatrists have personalities just like everyone else, and some are more prone to worry about potential litigation, while others are not.

For psychiatrists, the most common cause of litigation is a patient suicide. In any setting, it is terribly distressing, even devastating, when a patient dies from suicide. Suicide prevention efforts are a common focus of care, and psychiatrists routinely do risk assessments. No one would question that this is a worthwhile effort, and it certainly affects the business of psychiatry. Because of the fear of patient suicide, doctors may lower their threshold for hospitalization or may increase the frequency of patient appointments. Psychiatrists also think about the physical environment, for example, by modifying windows so they can't open from the inside or installing breakaway shower rods in an inpatient unit.

Fortunately, patient violence is rare; but it is a potential cause of litigation and can affect the financial aspect of any mental health system. This was not an issue for Sharon, but it had been for Mitchell, the patient in the last chapter, when he became agitated while in the hospital. Special precautions are needed in any setting where violence may occur. These patients are more expensive to care for because they require extra security services and precautions. In emergency departments and inpatient settings, patients may be very ill and unpredictable. Security measures may include extra staff, seclusion rooms, special call buttons, and even metal detectors. Although actual workplace violence is unusual—that is, violence against the psychiatrist in his office—psychiatrists do sometimes work with patients who have histories of assault, are perpetually bad tempered, or are at risk of being violent again. In this situation, a common business practice is to develop a behavior plan, or contract, that the patient must agree to as a condition of treatment.

Severe sociopaths who are at high risk for violence are usually treated in a secure setting such as a prison. Behavior contracts are not necessary in this setting because the institution itself has documented rules and consequences for violent behavior. When a threat occurs, the doctor weighs the seriousness of the threat and the reason for it. A patient might be blowing off steam and merely venting frustration by saying something threatening on an impulse. If the patient actually loses his temper or appears to be on the verge of losing behavioral control, the psychiatrist would respond by calling the patient's attention to his temper and offering to end the appointment. Sometimes the inmate himself will end the appointment and leave the office, or ask to return to his cell, to avoid acting out. Extra precautions are often taken for the next appointment, and a psychologist may be asked to attend the session for the sake of having another person in the room, or a correctional officer may remain outside the door (out of earshot) during the appointment. Certainly, in these settings, the cost of psychiatric care must include many security measures at considerable expense to the penal system.

What happens when a patient is actually violent in the context of care: when he meaningfully threatens or assaults his psychiatrist? It's not unheard of for patients to kill their psychiatrists, but fortunately, this is an extremely rare event. Patients can be combative, and in the course of their agitation, they can threaten members of their treatment team, or even assault them. This is the biggest intrusion on treatment, and events such as serious threats or an actual attack nearly always end treatment with that doctor. A therapeutic relationship can only work if both the patient and the doctor feel safe. The patient is also subject to consequences if he is threatening or violent. In a correctional facility this can include being written up and put on disciplinary segregation, as well as a longer sentence for the prisoner if the assault results in a new criminal charge. In a community setting, the clinician may decide to press criminal charges, and a patient may be forbidden from receiving further care at that site. A violent patient can be discharged from an inpatient unit or transferred to a more secure setting such as a forensic hospital. The final disposition often depends on the patient's condition and whether the violence is seen as a product of disturbed thinking or of bad behavior. A patient who is delusional and becomes combative because of his illness will be managed quite differently from a patient who is angry about the institutional rules.

We are mentioning the issue of violence because office policies sometimes include conditions that would cause a psychiatrist to discharge a patient from care. In addition to violent behavior, failure to pay for services may lead to discharge from treatment. Institutions may have specific rules about this, and the doctor may not have any input about whether a patient is discharged. A patient who has been treated in a publicly funded clinic may no longer be eligible for services there if she obtains private health insurance. This may be indicative of the patient's recovery, for example, when a previously unemployed patient gains health insurance as a benefit of a new job. In some cases, this happy event may be tainted by the sadness that a successful therapeutic relationship must end.

"I can't come anymore," Sharon said.

"Oh?" her doctor asked. Sharon was doing well in treatment. She'd gained twelve pounds and developed much healthier habits. Still, she was struggling with the idea that she was fat, and she was working on several important issues in therapy. She wasn't ready to stop treatment.

"My husband was laid off at work," she said. "We lose our health insurance at the end of the month, and I'm worried about paying the bills."

In private practices, doctors vary in how they handle changes in the patient's ability to pay; some continue seeing patients who can no longer pay, but others do not. Many factors come into play here, including the doctor's financial circumstances as well as his personal feelings about the patient and her treatment. Perhaps a patient has been particularly difficult to treat—for example, the patient misses appointments, will not take the medications the doctor recommends, is often argumentative, or frustrates the psychiatrist. Or perhaps the patient is financially strapped because of poor choices, not hard luck. A psychiatrist may not feel a desire to extend charity to a patient who is in financial straits because of careless spending on luxury items. In Sharon's case, they discussed the options, and she decided to come less often until her financial situation was stabilized. Her doctor told her she could make payments when she was able, but he did not offer to see her for a reduced rate.

Sharon talked to her doctor about all the stress she was experiencing at home and at work.

"Sam is home all day, but he doesn't lift a finger. I'm at work all day, then I come home and clean up after him. I have trouble falling asleep at night, and during the day, I'm anxious about whether or not Sam is going to find another job."

Sharon's doctor recommended she temporarily take a small dose of medicine for sleep and anxiety.

"Is it expensive?" she asked.

"Not at all," said her doctor. "I've got some samples I can give you for free. You'll only need it temporarily, so I won't have to write a prescription."

The pharmaceutical industry also exerts an influence on the business of psychiatry in obvious and in subtle ways. In addition to developing new medications, the industry influences how these medications are prescribed. Pharmaceutical marketing has been shown to influence how doctors prescribe certain medications through their relationships with pharmaceutical salespeople, also known as drug reps.

Drug companies spend tens of billions of dollars in marketing their products to physicians and in educating them about the benefits of the drugs. Drug reps used to drive home their points by leaving office products with the name and logo of the medication—sticky pads, pens, clipboards, coffee mugs, clocks, calendars, and so forth. The industry recently agreed to stop leaving these tchotchkes because such marketing tactics may unduly influence physician decisions, possibly resulting in the unnecessary prescription of a new and expensive drug over a less expensive alternative. They have also largely stopped doing the more blatant advertising activities that occurred in the past, such as educational cruises where the programs were focused on presenting evidence in support of the wonders of their products. Some of these changes have come about because drug companies have been criminally prosecuted for illegal marketing activities, and questionable marketing practices have caught the attention of federal agencies.

Physicians may feel that they are not influenced by token marketing gifts, but these freebies may create a sense of obligation to return the favor in some manner. Would Sharon's doctor have considered another medication if he hadn't had samples? Possibly. Most physicians would not consciously accept such a "bribe" in return for writing prescriptions for a particular product, so the industry learned how to manipulate physicians to do this in an unconscious manner. Now, many of these psychological marketing techniques are not allowed, and when pharmaceutical companies sponsor events, they are mandated to clearly state that sponsorship. In many settings, pharmaceutical representatives are no longer welcome because of concerns that these relationships are not ethical. The American Medical Association's ethical standards for physicians advise against doctors accepting gifts, and some academic centers are also developing guidelines to address physician-industry collaboration.

Instead, the drug industry now markets directly to consumers, called DTC marketing. The companies' advertisements must be approved by the FDA or they face stiff fines. Ads can be used only to market for medication uses that have FDA approval, and the ads must also list the more common side effects of a medication. Such ads steer treatment in that patients request very specific medications from physicians in a way we have not seen in the past. The ads may also destigmatize the treatment of mental illness because psychiatric illnesses are depicted only as medical constellations of symptoms with effective treatments.

Pharmaceutical companies have been major sponsors of research and have helped develop new and innovative treatments. Unfortunately, such sponsorship has not been untainted. When we learn that key investigators were paid huge sums of money to give talks on the value of a medication and that their studies promote the widespread use of a drug, it sullies the reputation of both the investigator and the drug company and brings into question the validity of the research. Such relationships may corrupt the research that we've been so eager to trust. In addition, pharmaceutical companies have not always been forthcoming about letting doctors or the public know about some of the harmful effects of their medications, which has resulted in class action litigation. These problems are not limited to psychiatry. When the integrity of the pharmaceutical companies and the research they support gets called into question, the public, understandably, may be less likely to try medications.

Has the pendulum swung too far in the other direction? In an effort to be certain that pharmaceutical companies no longer intrude on treatment, many institutions have severed ties with pharmaceutical companies. Pharmaceutical sales representatives are no longer allowed to visit many clinics for fear that any impropriety may be inferred. As a result, many institutions are no longer accepting samples of expensive medications. These samples have been crucial to providing the newest medications to indigent patients who have no means of paying for them. It remains unclear how the end of medication sampling will intrude on care. Also, the educational programs that were sponsored by pharmaceutical companies were often very helpful for teaching physicians about new treatments. It seems odd to ban pharmaceutical salespeople from educating physicians about their products, while direct-to-consumer advertisements—complete with attractive actors and minimal information—is considered a proper way to promote new treatments.

Sharon came to her appointment one day with slices of homemade cake.

"I want you to have this," she said.

"Did you eat any?" the doctor asked, with a smile. Sharon loved to cook and bake, but only for others. For herself, she worried about the calories.

"Actually, I did," she said. "And I wanted to bring you something because you've been so nice about letting me wait to pay you."

Pharmaceutical companies give doctors "gifts" to encourage sales of their products. But what about personal gifts from patients? Do these "buy" a therapist's favor? Psychiatric services are rendered in exchange for professional fees. Other gifts, particularly expensive gifts or those of an intimate nature, constitute a boundary transgression.

Different psychiatrists feel differently about accepting gifts: some simply refuse them, while others worry that it's hurtful to reject a gift, so they accept presents from patients. Unlike internists who may routinely accept holiday offerings or gifts given out of gratitude, most psychiatrists feel uneasy about accepting presents. The traditional psychiatric teaching is that it's wrong to accept a gift and that the offer of a gift should be an issue for therapeutic exploration. What does it mean to the patient to give the gift to the therapist? What does it mean if the doctor does or doesn't accept it? Obviously, there are no simple answers to these questions because the meaning varies for each patient and each psychiatrist as well as for the context in which it is offered. A patient's invitation to spend a weekend on his yacht is a completely different issue from a plate of homemade cookies brought in during the holiday season.

Even something as simple as a plate of holiday cookies can be handled in various ways. The doctor may feel comfortable receiving them from one patient (especially if the doctor likes cookies and the patient is a pastry chef) and uncomfortable receiving them from another patient, for example, one who has paranoid delusions about being poisoned and has difficulties maintaining a reasonable standard of personal hygiene. And the psychiatrist might feel uneasy at the next session if the patient asks how he liked the cookies and he hadn't eaten them, even if for personal reasons such as having diabetes or being allergic to nuts—facts he may not wish to share with his patients.

Sometimes, the therapeutic exploration gets uncomfortable, especially if the patient is not curious about her motives. As with asking a patient to explore why she's chronically late or repeatedly cancels appointments on short notice, the psychiatrist may feel that it is socially inappropriate to inquire about the patient's deeper motives for offering a holiday gift or a token of appreciation as therapy is ending.

For many psychiatrists, the issue of accepting gifts remains a bit awkward, and it is certainly considered wrong for a doctor to welcome presents of significant monetary value. This is not to say that psychiatrists don't like expressions of gratitude (or cookies!). Doctors usually enjoy hearing that they've been helpful to patients, and psychiatrists are no exception. Does a token gift affect care? As with most of the things we've discussed, we're left to say that it may or may not, in a good way or bad, depending on the complexities of the relationship between that particular psychiatrist and that particular patient.

Although we wish psychiatrists could simply treat patients and provide the best care without consideration of money, litigation, patient and staff safety, or practice management issues, this isn't the current reality of any mental health system. We hope that this open discussion of the issues will at least lead to a better understanding of what goes into our work.

Sharon did well in treatment. She never stopped worrying about her weight, but she stopped starving herself and developed healthier habits. She used therapy effectively, and she took medications just briefly. She was able to get the family health insurance through her employer, and six months later, her husband started a new job.

Chapter 11

Things We Argue About

UP TO NOW, we've used fictional patients to talk about psychiatry. In this chapter, we discuss topics that don't directly involve the relationship between doctor and patient, topics that can't be easily illustrated by an invented character. This chapter covers some of the controversies in our field.

Psychiatry is a uniquely controversial medical field. The question has been raised as to whether mental illness even exists, or if the disorders we treat simply represent variations of normal characteristics along the wide spectrum of emotions, reactions, and behaviors that human beings exhibit. We have floundered in our efforts to classify disorders, and many say that psychiatry has pathologized everything from routine discomfort to bad behavior. We have no definitive blood tests or x-rays to confirm any of our diagnoses, and the efficacy of our treatments has been questioned. While our efforts have brought us closer to consensus about what treatments work for what problems, we still have a long way to go.

Psychiatrists agree on a few things: we all agree that mental illness exists and that some of our treatments help some of our patients some of the time. It's hard enough that those outside our field express skepticism, if not anger, and often pass judgment on our patients, who come looking for help, and on those of us who try to help them; but among ourselves, we disagree about some very basic issues in our field. We disagree about how to distribute care in a world with limited resources, about how psychiatric diagnoses are defined, and about who deserves special considerations and financial support because of their illnesses. We do not have a

consensus about the role of addictive medications and alternative therapies in the treatment of psychiatric diseases. And finally, we don't have a
consensus about how to respond to those who have unified against our
field.

As this book was being written, health care reform became a reality in
this country. If ever there was a topic to argue about, this was it—and not
just for psychiatrists! Congress passed a health care bill designed to ex-
pand coverage to millions of uninsured Americans. We hope this will be
good news for poor or chronically mentally ill patients who have not had
insurance coverage. Often these patients get care only through emergency
rooms or correctional facilities. They may have difficulty getting care
outside these settings because they can't pay for it, or because the demand
for services is so great that they must wait weeks, or even months, for an
appointment. Our health system has been skewed in inconsistent and
unfair ways. The wealthy can choose concierge medical services, people
who work full time are often eligible for health insurance through their
employers, and some members of our population are eligible for Medicare and Medicaid. Others simply have no access to health insurance and
no money to pay for services. People who have been incarcerated are
frequently among the most vulnerable; their criminal records make it
difficult for them to obtain employment, and their finances are often
limited. Our current system has many inequities, and the uninsured patient does not fare well. We hope that health care reform will help narrow
the gap between the haves and the have-nots.

It would seem logical for physicians to be uniformly in favor of reform, but concerns about increased oversight and fear of governmental
intrusion in health care decisions, as well as the possibility of decreased
reimbursement, leave us torn.

It was difficult enough to get a health care reform bill passed, and the
implementation of new policy is certain to lead to even more arguments.
As more people have access to care, we may need to decide how to allocate our health care resources. Who decides if a condition requires treatment? Should we use a medical necessity standard, and how would we
define what exactly that means? Should elective procedures also be covered? What about experimental or unproven treatments? Should patients
get all the care they demand or only the care they "need"? And should

the physician be the gatekeeper, the one making the decision about how much care a patient should receive? The physician's obligation to offer the best possible care to his patient may clash with a societal obligation to limit medical spending. Our society retains the right to decide who is a patient—whether they want to be or not—through the use of civil commitment and involuntary treatment. Should society therefore also retain the right to decide who isn't a patient—those whose conditions are so advanced that treatment is futile, or so minor that treatment is unnecessary? These aren't new issues, but we may be hearing much more about them as changes are implemented.

In psychiatry, allocation concerns often revolve around specific treatments, and psychiatrists don't all value the same therapeutic modalities. Medications can be very expensive, particularly newer antipsychotic medications. Insurance companies, and public health care systems, want to contain the use of these medications since there are equally effective but less expensive medicines available. The controversy arises because the newer, more expensive medications have fewer side effects and are frequently tolerated better by patients.

Inpatient hospitalization is strongly influenced by managed care agencies that require justification in return for payment for admission and for continued inpatient treatment. Psychotherapy has also been limited by insurance companies that cover only a certain number of sessions, or by their managed care companies, which require preapproval and proof of medical necessity before they will reimburse for those sessions. Psychiatrists share some of these issues with other medical doctors. Insurance companies have formularies—lists of medicines they will cover—and discourage inpatient care for every specialty. Putting limits on outpatient care, however, is unique to psychiatry. If a patient has abdominal pain, he can schedule appointments with his physician as often as he wants (or as often as his doctor will have him!), without being preapproved by an insurance company.

No one would suggest that a patient who is suicidal should be denied care, or that disorganized and dangerous behavior isn't a reason to seek treatment. But psychiatric illness can be episodic, and receiving care during periods when symptoms have subsided may prevent future episodes of illness in some individuals. Regular monitoring also allows psychiatrists to catch episodes early, before a full-blown and disabling relapse. Patients who have been treated for cancer are often asked to have expensive diagnostic studies at regular intervals after treatment, even if they have no symptoms, with the hope that catching a new tumor early will improve the prognosis. Unlike with cancer patients, however, we have not yet figured out when a psychiatric patient may officially be declared "free" of disease so that monitoring can be stopped. These issues can be difficult to quantify, and health care systems will likely continue to establish boundaries for treatment in areas where research is unclear or lacking. Whether health care should be aimed toward maximizing the health of each individual, or toward maximizing the health of society as a whole, remains a difficult question.

Some psychiatrists favor health care reform and would like to see a single-payer system. Others worry that such a system would not pay for the treatments our patients need. Psychiatrists don't always agree on exactly what is needed—can a patient be maintained on medications alone with infrequent visits, or is psychotherapy also necessary? Some psychiatrists believe that the most expensive treatments should be limited to those with severe mental illnesses, while others favor treatment for everyone who requests it.

Physicians are concerned that under health care reform, they will lose autonomy over their practices. Patients are concerned that they will not be allowed to have the degree of care they want, or will lose health care choices. In fact, both parties have a role to play in health care cost containment, and many questions remain as Barack Obama's new health care system evolves. Both psychiatrists and patients are facing a future in which treatment, although—we hope—more equitable, will also be accompanied by some degree of anxiety. Clearly, these are provocative issues, and even the three of us don't agree.

Psychiatrists also disagree on which symptoms and behaviors should be classified as mental illnesses. It should be simple, but it isn't. The American Psychiatric Association's *Diagnostic and Statistical Manual* (DSM) is now going into its fifth edition. It has been a long process, over many years, to determine what is a psychiatric illness and what is not, and these categories are re-examined every decade or two. The decision to call a condition a disorder is determined by the consensus of a committee after much discussion, review of the research, input from experts, and opinions imposed from inside and outside the field. Many agendas are at work here. Patient advocacy groups may want their members to receive the allowances that a diagnosis might carry, while other advocacy groups do not want their members labeled in a way they feel is derogatory. One group favors inclusion of a disorder in the DSM, and another group opposes inclusion of the same disorder. The pharmaceutical industry may also have reasons to support certain diagnoses because it gives them a basis for marketing treatments. While psychiatrists may have their own views about diagnostic entities, if every emotion and every behavior were seen as "normal," we'd be out of a job.

The issue of diagnostic accuracy is important for research purposes. It is essential that a study of treatments for schizophrenia, for example, include only individuals who suffer from that particular illness. In clinical practice, diagnosis is used to guide treatment and can be used for prognosis. Patients and their families want to know what to expect over time, and the hope is that accurate diagnosis might help us see a bit into the future. Sometimes it works that way, and sometimes it doesn't. We are still not very good at accurately predicting who will do well and under what conditions, and who will be plagued by a lifetime of distress.

What's the controversy? Our diagnostic criteria for major mental illnesses seem like a Chinese menu: if you have two symptoms from column A and three symptoms from column B, and they've lasted a certain amount of time and can't be explained by another diagnosis or cause, then you have Disorder X. And actually, over time, we've come to reasonable agreement about many major mental illnesses. But sometimes the diagnosis is not as simple as defining symptoms. For example, in early editions of DSM, such as DSM-II, homosexuality was deemed a psychiatric disorder. It is now considered to be a variation in human attraction, and not a psychiatric disease. It wasn't that we originally believed that people with homosexual attractions had a difference in their blood levels or brain scans or anything else that we could measure, and that we discovered this is not, in fact, true. It's not even that all human beings agree now on whether homosexuality represents a disorder. But as our cultural beliefs about homosexuality have changed, the members of the task force that write the DSM reconsidered the decision to deem homosexuality a psychiatric illness.

The decision process is not very medical, and interest groups will lobby for or against the addition of a condition into the *Diagnostic and Statistical Manual*. Psychiatrists, too, will have views about what is and isn't a legitimate disorder that should or should not be the focus of treatment. An individual psychiatrist's views can be influenced by many things, including her personal and religious beliefs, what she was taught during training, her own clinical observations, and what she has learned from the research.

We know from epidemiological studies that some disorders have a genetic basis. We know that someone will have an increased risk of developing schizophrenia if he has a close relative with schizophrenia, even if he is raised by an adoptive family far away from any environmental influences. Similarly, people with borderline personality disorder tend to have relatives with bipolar disorder, indicating some type of genetic association between the two categories of illness. Even other personality disorders are likely to have a familial basis; people with antisocial personality disorder tend to have relatives with the disorder, though we certainly don't yet know if that is purely genetic or a result of a shared environment.

One frustration of psychiatric diagnosis is that whether a condition "counts" as a disorder depends on the context and culture in which the diagnosis is made. Social anxiety disorder may be disabling for some people, but others contend that it is simply a variant of "shyness," and that the creation of the diagnosis attempts to turn a human trait into pathology. It also allows pharmaceutical companies to market medications to treat the disorder. When it comes to reimbursement for treatment by insurance companies, some conditions are not considered valid as a focus of treatment, and these diagnoses will not be paid for. Substance abuse and dependence do not "count" as reasons for a psychiatric admission, and psychiatric hospitals are not typically reimbursed for inpatient care unless the person has an additional psychiatric disorder. Similarly, personality disorders can cause tremendous distress and dysfunction, but insurance companies will generally not pay for treatment—either inpatient or outpatient—unless there is another diagnosis. The presence or absence of a given diagnosis may determine whether an individual will qualify for certain jobs or programs or receive disability payments, or whether doctors will be paid for working with that patient. In extreme situations, a psychiatric "diagnosis" can be used as an avenue of repression. In the 1970s and 1980s, political dissidents in the Soviet Union were confined to psychiatric hospitals for behaviors such as distributing political propaganda or promoting religious freedom.

Are psychiatric diagnoses being stretched to cover a political or social need? Are diagnoses being created purely for the financial gain of people who treat the condition? Or for the pharmaceutical companies that manufacture medications to manage these new disorders? One example is the diagnosis "paraphilia, not otherwise specified," which is found in DSM-IV. This diagnosis is frequently given to exhibitionists or criminals convicted of repeated rapes. Many insurance companies do not reimburse clinicians for treatment of disorders related to criminal behavior, and this may limit treatment options. For the DSM-V, there is the proposed diagnosis of "paraphilic coercive disorder," a technical term for forcing someone to have sexual relations, or rape. The consideration of this behavior as a "new" disorder has caused a fair amount of controversy. Will someone with this condition be found insane? Will he be eligible for disability payments or workplace accommodation? Or is this just another way for a mental health clinician to get paid? Clearly, the intent is not to protect the rapist from prosecution or responsibility for his behaviors, yet it might be beneficial for someone to have a means to seek help before he acted on an impulse to commit a heinous act, or to get treatment during an incarceration to help prevent another such offense after release from prison.

Where do psychiatrists disagree? Certainly, we don't know any psychiatrists who believe that political dissidents should be confined to psychiatric hospitals, or that being intoxicated would be an excuse for harming another person. And there are certainly some diagnostic entities on which we all agree: the young person who hears voices and has delusions is clearly ill, as is the woman who can't get out of bed and thinks only of taking her own life. But sometimes even trained psychiatrists don't agree on what a normal reaction to a difficult situation looks like, or whether certain psychiatric entities even exist.

Some examples of diagnostic disagreement in psychiatry include our use of the diagnoses of bipolar disorder and of dissociative identity disorder. Over time, we've broadened our conception of bipolar disorder to include milder episodes of mood elevation and states of irritability in a way that previously would not have been captured by this diagnosis. Our understanding of this illness in children and adolescents is still being defined. Many people, including psychiatrists, feel that bipolar disorder is diagnosed too easily in too many people and is a label that is sometimes given to people with bad behavior or those who are facing difficult developmental challenges. The popular press is quick to say that medications are overprescribed for those who are not truly ill. Some psychiatrists believe this is true, while others feel these illnesses have gone unnoticed and untreated in many people for far too long.

Many psychiatrists believe that the symptom constellation previously called multiple personality disorder (now renamed dissociative identity disorder) can be explained by other diagnostic categories such as a personality disorder, or bipolar disorder, or a severe form of anxiety. We talked about this in chapter 6 when Becca Brandt was told she had several different personalities. It leaves us with the question of who is right, if anyone, about the validity of this diagnostic category. There will likely be many more versions of the DSM as our knowledge about the biology of psychiatric disorders grows and our cultural values evolve.

A psychiatric diagnosis is a double-edged sword. Many people resent being labeled and feel that a mental illness may convey a dismal prognosis or limit their lives in several ways. Some patients are simply insulted by the idea that they are anything other than normal and well-adjusted. On the other hand, insurance companies reimburse for treatment only if a diagnosis is made, and our society makes certain allowances for people with handicaps, including mental illness, so a diagnosis can be helpful.

Psychiatrists are often involved in helping patients to obtain benefits because of psychiatric impairments, and this is another area on which we don't always agree. One of the allowances we make is to award disability payments to those who are too ill to work, including those who are too ill because of psychiatric disorders. The relationship between mental illness and the ability to work is not always clear. It is obvious that a person who has lost his legs can no longer perform certain jobs, but psychiatric symptoms are often not visible. In addition, symptoms of illness can be difficult to distinguish from laziness or a poor work ethic, or simply a person's desire to escape from a specific situation if she doesn't enjoy her work or has trouble with a boss or co-worker. It can be hard to know when people can't work versus when they won't work, and there is not always a correlation between the severity of symptoms and the ability to be employed. Some patients may be disabled even though they do not have active symptoms of illness and their medications are working. Perhaps they have only brief periods of stability and are unable to function reliably enough to maintain a job. Some psychiatric conditions decrease a person's motivation. On the other hand, some people are able to work despite very severe psychiatric symptoms. We don't have good ways of determining who exactly can work and who can't, and sometimes it is difficult to articulate exactly why it is that someone cannot maintain employment. Ultimately, the decision about who gets disability benefits is left to a governmental agency, with input from psychiatrists.

To add to the issue, if a person is able to work, it is often in his best interest to do so. Certainly, self-esteem is improved when one contributes to society, life is more fun with more money, and work adds a natural structure to a person's day in a way that is helpful. Once a person is declared disabled and entitled to long-term financial benefits, either Social Security income (SSI) or Social Security disability income (SSDI), then recovery and a return to work often mean losing those benefits. It often takes a long time, and the assistance of a lawyer, to get benefits, and few patients are willing to risk losing them by trying to return to full-time employment.

From a psychiatrist's point of view, disability payments may be both good and bad—they may help those with severe illnesses to maintain housing and nutrition and to get health care, but they may also promote a degree of dependence that is not necessary or even desirable for every patient requesting these benefits. Since we've been discussing fairness, it seems reasonable to comment that the allocation of disability benefits does not always make sense to us; sometimes very ill people are denied when those with less disabling symptoms are granted benefits. Among ourselves, we don't always agree on who is disabled and who is not.

Mental illness can cause difficulty getting or keeping a job. While the Americans With Disabilities Act bars discrimination based on psychiatric disorders, discrimination is notoriously hard to prove, and stigma is still very real in the workplace. To be protected by the ADA, the job applicant must make his disability known to the potential employer and must be otherwise able to perform the duties and responsibilities of the job. If both of these conditions are met, employers are required to make reasonable accommodation for the disabled worker. The definition of "reasonable" has been a source of litigation for a while now, but for physical illnesses, it usually means allowing the worker to bring in, or use, adaptive devices like back supports, wrist braces, wheelchairs, or crutches. It also may mean reassignment of nonessential duties, allowance for frequent breaks to take medication or monitor a symptom, or leave allowance to attend medical appointments. For mentally ill workers, reasonable accommodation could mean modifying the work environment to minimize interruptions and decrease distracting noise, or allowing workers to take time for psychiatric appointments. Some employees have been allowed flexible work schedules. In practice, most workers with psychiatric disorders do not ask for, or need, special accommodations on the job, and their most common request is for time off when they have an episode of illness.

While the intention of the ADA is to allow those with disabilities more access to jobs, the down side is that mandating accommodation may inadvertently increase the stigma of having a mental illness by implying that psychiatric patients need a leg up compared with others and are incapable of competing on a level playing field. People vary a great deal in terms of how much mental illness affects their ability to work, and many people feel it is in their best interest to conceal their psychiatric diagnoses from their employers. There are times, however, when illnesses interfere with work, and legal protections may allow patients with psychiatric disabilities to maintain employment.

Vocational rehabilitation services are available to those with illnesses. These services may include job coaching, vocational skills assessment, and referrals to supported employment opportunities. These opportunities allow people with chronic and severe illnesses to work in environments that are more sheltered than a competitive workplace, though they do not typically pay as much. Many of these programs are designed so that patients can work part time and earn some income without losing their SSDI payments.

The situation becomes more complicated when people with psychiatric disorders request accommodation that is unusual or that may intrude on the comfort of others, and this brings us back to the issues psychiatrists disagree about. For example, the airlines have begun to allow passengers to travel with support animals. Often these are dogs, but other animals are also used. The passenger must present a physician's letter stating that the animal is needed to help during the flight or with activities at the destination. These animals are typically used by patients with anxiety problems, but they do become a public announcement of sorts that a problem exists for the owner. The animals are usually trained and well behaved, and the question might be raised as to why this would present a problem, or why everyone can't travel with a dog. In general, the presence of a trained support animal is not a problem, but what happens if the passenger in the next seat is allergic to animal fur, is phobic of dogs, or simply doesn't want to be near a dog (especially one with a small bladder) on the plane? The issue can become a battle over whose rights are more valid. According to articles in the *New York Times*, the use of emotional support animals on airplanes has been stretched to include support ducks and goats! We are not likely to come to a consensus about the role psychiatrists should play in asserting that patients need to fly with their animals.

These issues of special accommodation are not unique to those with psychiatric disorders. For example, educators give extra time on college entrance exams to those students who've been diagnosed with learning disabilities. Sometimes these learning impairments are subtle and require extensive (and expensive) testing for diagnosis—a process that is more readily available to those who can afford to pay for it. Another example, also with the airlines, includes the question of what is reasonable when seating morbidly obese passengers. Should they be charged for two seats or permitted to buy just one ticket, even if this leaves the people in adjacent seats with less room? There are many ways in which our society struggles with issues of fairness.

In addition to increasing stigma, another risk of accommodation is that the accommodation itself may encourage patients to consider themselves lesser individuals. In general, we don't want to encourage people to be victims when they could simply be people with differences.

What about sensitive jobs in which the symptoms of a mental disorder could affect the lives or safety of others? Should a person with a mental illness be allowed to be president or governor? These issues are repeatedly raised in the media. And what about a soldier or police officer who must carry a weapon? Certainly if the person is symptomatic, this is cause for alarm. Mental illness can cause poor judgment, suicidal thoughts, and slow reaction times. But what if the officer hasn't been ill for a long time? What about politicians who control national defense? Should every presidential candidate have a psychiatric evaluation before throwing a hat into the ring? Thomas Eagleton, a vice-presidential candidate in 1972, chose to withdraw from the race when it was publicized that he had a history of depression and had been treated with electroconvulsive therapy. Was this reasonable?

The Federal Aviation Administration sets standards for the types of medications that pilots are allowed to take, and psychiatric medications are not allowed. As this chapter was being written, the FAA was considering a policy change regarding pilots who take antidepressants. The new policy would allow pilots to fly while being treated for depression, but only after twelve months of satisfactory treatment and only after being given a waiver to fly by an FAA-certified physician. If a pilot cannot be treated with medications without leaving his job, we're left to wonder if this doesn't encourage unstable pilots to hide their difficulties and fly untreated, a scenario that might be far more dangerous than having a pilot who is well on a medication. Ironically, pilots are allowed to take blood thinners or anti-arrhythmic medications even though the underlying medical conditions these medications treat can put them at risk of stroke or sudden death. When it comes to fitness for duty, mental disorders appear to be arbitrarily targeted over medical disorders. And psychiatrists don't always agree on what constitutes a risk to the public or what our role should be in advocating for our patients versus protecting society from potential risks, especially when these risks seem, to us, both minimal and unpredictable.

Some positions—for example, law enforcement professions—require psychiatric evaluations as part of a conditional job offer, but the presence of a psychiatric disorder does not bar employment if the individual is reasonably accommodated and can do the job. The trick with psychiatric disorders is that they are unpredictable, and people can suddenly get them for the first time, or have relapses at unexpected times, even with treatment. We need to have provisions for these events, and we need to have procedures to monitor the people involved. A diagnosis of anything should not, in and of itself, prevent someone from taking on a high-responsibility position. The question should be about how the person is currently functioning. And if a position carries enough high risk, for example, a nuclear weapons specialist or an airline pilot, then there should be built-in safeguards that require ongoing assessment of functional capacity, regardless of the presence or absence of diagnostic labels. One point seems clear, and that is if you take away someone's job simply because he seeks treatment, then people don't get care, and this may not be in the best interest of anyone.

What about the president of the United States? In current practice, the medical records of presidential candidates are reviewed not only by their personal physicians, but also by specific members of the media. We all agree that someone with such power and the ability to change history on an impulse should be a fast thinker with excellent judgment. The president should not be someone with a labile internal state that might influence his decisions, and the president should have an emotionally stable advisory staff. Have all our presidents been mentally well? A historical review of presidential biographies to 1974 revealed that 49 percent of past presidents have suffered from psychiatric disorders, including bipolar disorder, major depression, alcohol abuse, dependence on pain killers, sleep apnea, and anxiety. Some think that it is not likely that a president would be elected now if there was a known history of significant psychiatric disorder. Psychiatrists have different views on this, and the argument includes questions about what the disorder is, how severe or disabling the symptoms have been, how well the person is responding to treatment, and the likelihood of recurrence. When it comes to politics, the acceptance of a psychiatric condition is one that gets decided by the voters, or perhaps by the advisers who screen the candidates.

In addition to issues of diagnosis and accommodation, psychiatrists also argue about treatments. In chapter 5, we talked about the pros and cons of using Xanax, a medication that helps anxiety but is very addictive. Some of the medications we use in psychiatry are known as controlled substances: they have the potential to be addictive, and Xanax is just one of them. The most commonly prescribed addictive medications are the benzodiazepines, including Librium and Valium, which have been on the market since the early 1960s. These medications are used to treat many conditions, including anxiety, insomnia, agitation, panic attacks, seizures, spasticity, restless leg syndrome, and alcohol withdrawal. They are also used for sedation before medical procedures. What's nice is that they work very soon after they are taken; they don't need days or weeks to have a positive effect the way some other types of medicines do. They help with acute anxiety after a single dose, and they help with chronic anxiety if they are taken regularly. Valium was nicknamed—by the media, not by psychiatrists!—"mother's little helper," a name that trivializes the problems it was prescribed for, as well as the significant risks associated with it. Benzodiazepines did many good things, and in fact, they virtually replaced the dangerous and highly addictive barbiturates as the medication of choice for anxiety and sleep disorders. But, like barbiturates, benzodiazepines proved to be more habit-forming than initially recognized. In some patients, the medications led to tolerance, dependence, and difficulty coming off them.

Stimulants, such as Ritalin, are another class of medications that can lead to abuse, dependence, and addiction but that have therapeutic value and are often prescribed by psychiatrists to treat disorders of attention and hyperactivity, as well as depression and sleep disorders such as narcolepsy.

Psychiatrists agree that these medications can be helpful, and we agree that these medications can be addictive. What we don't agree on is whether the risk of addiction outweighs the benefits of addictive medications. In terms of the older barbiturates, the jury is in, and these medications are no longer used for psychiatric purposes. They remain useful as anesthetics for surgery and for the treatment of seizures, but they are too addictive, and too dangerous if taken incorrectly, to remain in use for general psychiatric purposes, especially now that we have safer and more effective treatments.

Prescribing controlled substances is challenging because psychiatrists don't always know, nor can we predict, which patients will develop dependency and addiction to these medications. Psychiatrists are not mind readers or lie detectors—it's difficult for doctors to know when someone is seeing a prescriber for the sole purpose of obtaining a controlled substance. And while controlled substances are useful for some conditions, the medications can also be easily diverted, that is, sold illegally or given away to others.

Often the prescribing physician is the last to know when his medication is being abused or diverted. Psychiatrists who work in correctional facilities frequently hear from their patients that they abused prescribed medications before they were incarcerated. Patients with a drug addiction will obtain controlled substances by visiting more than one doctor, or by sending a girlfriend to visit a doctor, or by taking medicine that was prescribed for someone else. People sometimes go to extreme measures to get addictive medications. While we commonly picture drug addicts as scruffy individuals making covert drug deals on the corner, some of those addicts started on the road to addiction with a legal prescription given for a legitimate pain or anxiety problem.

While psychiatrists agree that benzodiazepines can be helpful, we disagree on the circumstances in which they should be prescribed. Most psychiatrists would feel comfortable prescribing a controlled substance to a patient who has no history of addiction, for a limited time, as long as the patient was given informed consent about the risk. Some psychiatrists would use benzodiazepines to treat anxiety in a patient with a history of addiction to other substances, but only if the addiction was under control and the patient was in recovery, and if the patient was informed about the risk of benzodiazepine dependence. Other psychiatrists would not feel comfortable doing this even if the patient was in recovery.

Benzodiazepines can be used temporarily to help patients deal with anxiety until another medication can build up to therapeutic levels. They can be used on an as-needed basis for acute anxiety. Regular doses of benzodiazepines, taken several times a day, can be used to treat anxiety long term, and there are patients who've taken these medicines for decades. Among psychiatrists, we don't have a consensus on what is beneficial to any given patient or whether these medications are under- or overused. There are those who feel that these medicines create more problems than they cure, while others feel they are effective treatments that are unnecessarily withheld from patients when they could provide relief.

The issues are not much different with other habit-forming medications. Most psychiatrists do not prescribe narcotics, but those who specialize in pain management may use them in their practices. Psychiatrists, along with pediatricians, are often responsible for prescribing stimulants for attention deficit disorder. When a patient says a specific medication is the only thing that helps and is unwilling to explore other treatments, when he requests escalating doses, or when he loses prescriptions, red flags start to go up, and the doctor may consider drug abuse.

Marijuana is a legally prescribed medication in some states. It is not regulated by the FDA, and its efficacy has not been fully tested, but it has been legalized for the treatment of a host of conditions: nausea, fibromyalgia, weight loss associated with AIDS, chronic pain, gastrointestinal distress, multiple sclerosis, and other illnesses. Recently the American Medical Association recommended that marijuana be reclassified as a drug with possible medicinal benefits. It also called for more research to clarify the medicinal potential of the drug.

The use of marijuana in the treatment of psychiatric disorders is controversial because of its addictive nature but also because little clinical data support the efficacy of marijuana for many psychiatric conditions. In Colorado, each medical marijuana patient is registered; to date, nearly twenty thousand people are on the registry. Marijuana advocates have attempted to add anxiety and bipolar disorder to the list of conditions for which doctors can prescribe marijuana, but these efforts have failed due to lack of proven efficacy. There are anecdotes of patients who say it helps, but controlled studies have not been done.

If the use of benzodiazepines is controversial among psychiatrists, we anticipate that marijuana will be even more so. In states where marijuana laws have been liberalized, there has been an explosion of marijuana clinics. There will be increasing pressure on psychiatrists to prescribe, and each of us will have to make an individual decision. If the patient says it helps, should we prescribe it? What if there is little or no proven efficacy? What if the patient has a known history of addiction, regardless of her stage of recovery or abstinence from other substances? Will psychiatrists working in correctional facilities be required to continue marijuana prescribed by a free society doctor or risk litigation by refusing? Marijuana is a particularly controversial issue because it produces a high, and because it is associated with loss of motivation in some people. Decreased motivation is a difficult symptom to address and is frequently seen as a symptom of psychiatric disorders. As psychiatrists, we look for ways to help patients become motivated and to rely less on intoxicants. The issues, however, are much different when cannabis is taken in a pill form as Marinol or when it's used to treat nausea associated with cancer chemotherapy, a temporary condition, or anorexia associated with end-stage AIDS.

Controlled substances and addiction are a significant problem for society and individuals alike. Doctors must weigh patient risk factors against the legitimate and proven efficacy of each controlled substance and consider this information carefully in collaboration with the patient. This is an emerging area of medicine with no easy choices for psychiatrists.

There are many healing paradigms in the world, and traditional Western medicine is only one of them. Since psychiatry is a medical specialty, it is based on the principles of Western evidence-based medicine: randomized controlled trials, the scientific method, and measurable outcome data. In psychiatry, we encounter and explore other healing paradigms based on the culture and interests of the patients we treat. Psychiatrists vary in their level of acceptance of these alternative therapies and their willingness to work with patients who participate in them. Psychiatrists who strongly support unorthodox treatments risk being judged negatively by their colleagues and risk professional sanctions if patients complain that their care was compromised. This is one more area of disagreement in our field.

Psychiatrists support and encourage healthy lifestyle activities. Many patients participate in yoga, tai chi, and regular exercise. Regular physical activity helps mood, probably helps sleep, and certainly helps cardiac health. These activities are not typically promoted as mental health therapy, but there is little question that they are beneficial. Such activities are known as *complementary* because they add to, or augment, standard treatment, but they are generally not used as a sole intervention for serious mental disorders.

Alternative treatments, on the other hand, are those that are intended to be used alone, instead of standard Western medicine. Common types of alternative medicine are Ayurvedic or East Asian remedies, Chinese or Japanese herbal remedies, and nutritional supplements. The range of alternative medicinal products is so broad that we cannot cover each one individually. These treatments are not regulated by the FDA and are not subject to the rigors of research to clearly define their risks or benefits, much less their safety. One study of Ayurvedic remedies sold in New York City found that as many as one-fourth of them contained toxic heavy metals. Because the active ingredients of a pill aren't known, it's impossible to regulate the amount of herb that goes into each one, leading to variability among herbal preparations. And because many alternative remedies are manufactured overseas, their purity and content cannot be guaranteed.

The National Institutes of Health sponsors the National Center for Complementary and Alternative Medicine (NCCAM), the federal government's lead agency for scientific research on complementary and alternative medicine. NCCAM supports research on alternative treatments or therapies that are not considered part of conventional Western medicine. More information about some of them can be found on the NCCAM website at *http://nccam.nih.gov/research*.

Psychiatrists vary a great deal in terms of how much they encourage, support, or even tolerate the use of unproven treatments. Some doctors align themselves with providers of alternative and complementary treatments and encourage the use of acupuncture, supplements, and other holistic approaches. Others promote the use of conventional medication and dissuade patients from trying unproven treatments. What we do know is that treatments that are not marketed as medications are less stigmatized and may appeal to people who might hesitate to try psychiatric treatments. We also know that untested and unregulated therapies may be just as powerful as regular medicines, in both beneficial and dangerous ways.

Clearly, psychiatry has many areas of controversy, even from within, and even among the most influential thinkers in our field. What about controversy from outside? There are patients who feel they've been wronged by psychiatrists, by their diagnostic labels, and by adverse effects from medications and psychotherapy. There is a movement of individuals who have coalesced around the idea that psychiatry is harmful: the antipsychiatry movement. In addition to the assertion that psychiatry is ultimately more damaging than helpful to patients, the antipsychiatry movement calls attention to the imbalance of power between psychiatrists and their patients, and the demeaning nature of treatments that may require institutionalization, medication, and restriction of personal autonomy.

The antipsychiatry movement announces psychiatry's shortcomings, flaws, and mistakes. More recently, the *recovery model* has taken a consumer-oriented focus toward the treatment of patients. The recovery model emphasizes patient involvement in decisions, hopefulness, and movement toward individual empowerment and mental health.

Psychiatrists agree that treatments have been far from perfect, and that some treatments have terrible side effects. Historically, our field has struggled with how to best help patients within the context of our changing cultural values and the limited amount of evidence-based information we've had about what treatments might work. The antipsychiatry movement, boosted by the Church of Scientology's non-mainstream beliefs about mental illness (e.g., they refer to psychiatry as the "industry of death"), looks to portray psychiatrists as intentionally malevolent, rather than as physicians doing their best to help patients. Furthermore, former patients who feel they've been harmed by psychotropic medications may make public statements that all psychiatric medications are harmful and should be avoided by everyone under every condition. The antipsychiatry movement leaves very little room for individual differences.

In concert with society's shift away from paternalistic medicine, psychiatrists are more cognizant of giving patients informed consent about treatments and try not to make sweeping predictions about the course a patient's life will take after a diagnosis is made. The issue for both psychiatrists and for patients and their family members, however, becomes one of passing judgment. The recovery model is one in which semantics are very important—the term "patient" may be deemed demeaning, and the designation "consumer"—or even "ex-patient"—is preferred. Some people think that the model implies that everyone can be cured through sheer willpower and may blame the person with a disorder for not getting better. Another concern is that the model may be used for political and financial agendas to withdraw services from patients prematurely. And when a psychiatrist embraces the recovery model, there may be the hint of professional condemnation from other psychiatrists, an odd hint of collusion with the idea that past generations of psychiatrists have willfully wronged patients. In general, however, the idea that patients should actively participate in their treatment and should strive for a meaningful recovery from mental illness is one that our field should encourage.

Psychiatrists must be willing to acknowledge historical wrongs done by the profession while holding out hope that our treatments are, for the most part, beneficial. These issues demand a degree of open mindedness by both patients and doctors. We can't stress enough that each person is an individual, and though our science guides us toward answers for groups of people, the one-on-one interaction between a doctor and a particular patient may require something different or more.

Chapter 12

The Future of Psychiatry

PSYCHIATRISTS RELY ON medication to treat psychiatric diseases by altering brain neurochemistry. We rely on psychotherapy to help us treat problems related to difficult past events and relationships, and it, too, may alter the workings of the brain. We have strategies for dealing with conditions that resist the usual therapies. As we end our book, we'd like to talk about some of these experimental procedures in a little more detail and discuss some promising research for future psychiatric treatments.

In addition to medications, there are other ways of changing brain chemistry, and future psychiatrists may practice very differently than we do now with regard to diagnosing and treating mental disorders. We've talked about the limitations of our current diagnostic schemes and lamented the fact that we have no hard and firm diagnostic tests. Future psychiatrists may depend on genetic or imaging studies to diagnose disease and to design individualized treatments.

Many people are familiar with brain imaging studies like computer axial tomography (CT) scans and positron emission tomography (PET) scans, which take computer-enhanced pictures of the brain. Magnetic resonance imaging (MRI) studies can also take very detailed pictures by using a powerful magnetic field rather than x-rays. The latest incarnation of MRI is called functional magnetic resonance imaging, or fMRI. Functional MRI uses radio waves and a magnetic field to take detailed pictures and to measure metabolic changes in certain parts of the brain. Functional MRI studies are being used to clarify which parts of the brain are used for particular purposes by taking pictures while a person is doing a mental task, for example, looking at pictures or memorizing a list of words. This kind of research is called *brain mapping*.

Researchers are using mapping technology to figure out which parts of the brain are disturbed in patients with schizophrenia and to locate which specific regions are responsible for different symptoms. For example, fMRI has been used to show that people with schizophrenia mentally process auditory hallucinations in the same way that other people process language, even though the hallucinations aren't "real" sounds. Someday, perhaps, we'll be able to figure out who has schizophrenia and who has bipolar disorder just by taking a picture. This technology may also evolve to let people control computers by thought alone, which could help people with spinal cord injuries or neuromuscular diseases.

Functional MRI is being used to figure out the neuroanatomy behind risk-taking decisions, and even to determine when someone is lying. Clearly, this new technology has ethical and legal implications that society should prepare for. Will forensic psychiatrists one day be trained to interpret brain scans to decide legal issues like criminal insanity? Only time will tell.

Researchers are also studying new electromagnetic treatments for mental disorders. The three main new treatments are repetitive transcranial magnetic stimulation (rTMS), vagal nerve stimulation (VNS), and deep brain stimulation (DBS). Both VNS and DBS require surgical implantation of devices. While all these modalities are still in the experimental stage, some patients with treatment-resistant disease have experienced a degree of recovery.

Repetitive TMS has been used to treat tinnitus (chronic ringing in the ears), chronic pain, and clinical depression, and it is currently being used in clinical practice for treatment-resistant depression (i.e., that has not responded to medications). The treatment is thought to work by increasing metabolism in the parts of the brain involved in depression. The patient sees a psychiatrist who has an rTMS machine in the office and sits in a device that looks like a dental chair. Coils to generate a magnetic field are placed on the patient's head. In some cases, the coil position is determined by PET or MRI scan, to help identify poorly perfused areas of the brain. Some patients in research studies experienced as much as a 50 percent decrease in depressive symptoms. Right now, there aren't enough data to prove that rTMS is effective for any particular psychiatric disorder. Researchers disagree about where the leads should be placed, how long the stimulation should last, and how many treatments to give. Of course, any treatment that works also has potential risks. There have been case reports of rTMS causing mania and delusions.

VNS involves the surgical implantation of a small generator along with an electrode that intermittently stimulates a nerve that runs from the chest into the brain. The generator runs continuously, which means that the treatment is given constantly, sometimes for months or years. A small number of studies suggest that 10 to 30 percent of patients with treatment-resistant depression may have some response to this treatment. It has been approved by the FDA for use in depression, but only for patients who have not gotten better with four or more antidepressants. While there have been few documented side effects, some patients have had permanent changes in the quality of their voices. Temporary side effects include sore throat and neck stiffness.

DBS is the most invasive of the three electromagnetic treatments. Similar to VNS, a generator is implanted underneath the skin using a method similar to pacemaker placement. Then an electrode is implanted in a certain part of the brain, usually the subthalamic region. Deep brain stimulation has been used in Parkinson's disease and for the treatment of chronic pain. In psychiatry, DBS has been tried mainly for the treatment of severe obsessive-compulsive disorder (OCD) and, more rarely, treatment-resistant depression. A very small number of studies have shown up to 30 percent improvement in OCD symptoms. The results for depression are mixed and inconclusive due to the small number of studies. Of all the treatments discussed so far, DBS carries the most potentially serious side effects. Because the electrode must be planted directly in the brain, DBS carries the risk of brain hemorrhage, infection, and seizures.

All these electromagnetic therapies are based on the idea that the brain can grow and change and remodel itself, a process called *neuroplasticity*. The idea that the brain can change is a relatively new one. Once we thought that people were born with about a hundred billion nerve cells, or neurons, and that there could never be new ones. In fact, a large proportion of those neurons die off in the first six years of life, when a great deal of learning is going on. This cell death occurs not because of injury but as a result of a programmed process in the brain, during which the neurons that are used the most survive, while those that are just "sitting around" die off because they are not needed. Now we know that new neurons are created regularly, coming from stem cells inside the brain. This tends to happen more when damage has occurred, and the brain has to work around the damaged area, like a detour around an intersection because of construction work. It also occurs when new learning takes place. For example, if a person starts to learn to read Braille, the amount of brain area devoted to sensation in the fingertips expands greatly, even if that person isn't blind. Some of that may be due to new neurons but much is due to rewiring of the surrounding areas of the brain, to enlist more cells to help with the new endeavor of distinguishing the placement of raised dots on a piece of paper.

We are still learning the mechanisms involved in neuroplasticity. Drugs are being investigated that amplify or target this neuroplasticity, such that people with paralysis might be able to walk again. It turns out that people with depression have smaller hippocampi, which is the main memory area in the brain. It has been shown that the hippocampus loses brain cells during depression and that new brain cells grow as depression is successfully treated. Antidepressants cause new brain cells to grow, and this is one of the possible mechanisms by which these drugs improve depression. The promise of targeting the neuroplasticity functions of the brain is that we will someday be able to use the brain's own built-in repair mechanisms to fix problems that need more help than nature itself can resolve.

The idea of designing individualized treatment for each patient is called personalized medicine, sometimes referred to as genomic medicine. Genomic medicine is based on the idea that our DNA can give us a greater understanding of our various health risks and can help to better tailor treatments to the genetic makeup of the patient. Someday, if we have a large enough database of millions of peoples' DNA and their clinical history, we may discover combinations of clinical and genetic findings that predict a positive response to a certain drug. Personalized medicine promises to make this a reality. A good example of this is Roche's Amplichip P450. When this chip is exposed to a patient's DNA, a unique pattern of dots appears, each representing a certain genotype. The genes produce different liver enzymes, called P450 enzymes, which are responsible for breaking down various medications, including many of those used in psychiatry. This chip was approved by the FDA in 2005 for use as a method to better estimate how quickly people will metabolize medications to predict who will have side effects from different medications, including medications for depression, cancer, and cardiac conditions. As with many of the early promises of personalized medicine, the P450 chip has yet to gain widespread use in clinical practice. These tools are expected to be increasingly used in the future of medicine, but how long it will take is anybody's guess.

Currently drug companies develop and market drugs that help the widest swath of conditions, thus selling to a large market. As we learn more about the interaction between our genes, medications, and personal factors such as diet and exercise, the markets get split up into smaller and smaller segments. Someday we may see drug companies marketing to a subset such as "males under 30 with early onset, paranoid-type schizophrenia, who have a positive family history of schizophrenia, are responsive to the medication clozapine, have both of the short alleles for the 5HTT-linked polymorphism in the promoter region of the serotonin transporter (5-HTTLPR), and have a particular allele for the dopamine-3 receptor." This is a technical way of saying that we hope that one day we will be able to use each person's genetics to predict responses to medication.

None of these treatments is part of mainstream psychiatry, though rTMS is slowly becoming available to more patients. For now, these treatments are offered only to those who are desperate and a little bit courageous. What these new treatments suggest is that psychiatric researchers are approaching illness in many new and creative ways.

And what about psychotherapy? It has traditionally been the mainstay of psychiatric treatment, but in recent decades, psychotherapy has been less of an anchor in the care of patients, especially when that care is given by psychiatrists. While many psychiatrists still see patients for psychotherapy, many do not. Researchers continue to look at which forms of therapy are most effective for different conditions. Research aside, however, patients continue to say that psychotherapy is helpful. Part of the limitation of talk therapy is that we don't do an adequate job of articulating how and why it works, and it's become a treatment that is both difficult to learn and difficult to do. It's hard to imagine a future where psychiatry is simply about symptoms and side effects, however, with no curiosity about the emotional life of the person. We anticipate that psychotherapy will never become obsolete, and the pendulum may swing back toward emphasizing more thoughtful, human-based interventions with patients by psychiatrists, even as our biological treatments become more powerful.

This is an exciting time to be a psychiatrist. It is also a hopeful time for our patients. We wanted to share what we do in our work with patients, why we do it, and how we hope our work will help people to live more fulfilling lives. We hope you enjoyed reading about our professional lives as much as we enjoyed writing about them. Clearly, we're at the beginning of a long and eventful journey.

Acknowledgments

We would like to thank the many people who have helped us with this endeavor.

Our loved ones have been particularly patient as we've taken over the living space to produce dozens of podcasts, spent our time blogging and writing, and, at moments, loudly ranted at each other about psychiatric issues or simply the placement of a comma. For their love, support, inspiration, and encouragement, we'd like to thank David, Barb, Victor, Nathan, Donna, Rachel, and Jerry, not to mention the assorted pets who were displaced or secluded for our many meetings.

Dinah's sister-in-law Mary O'Keeffe, Ph.D., was invaluable as a reader who gave us an unbiased perspective and served as our representative of the lay audience interested in mental health issues we were planning to address. We couldn't have asked for a better reader and adviser.

The following friends and colleagues helped with the book in direct and time-consuming ways: Bruce Hershfield, M.D. (who sat with Dinah for hours and also brought fresh eggs), Jeffrey Janofsky, M.D., Emile Bendit, M.D., Christiane Tellefsen, M.D., Charles Jaffe, M.D., Elaine Tierney, M.D., Stuart Gitlow, M.D., and Scott Oakman, M.D. Without their help, this book would not have been possible. For the forensic chapters, we could have had no greater mentors and advisers than the faculty of the University of Maryland's forensic psychiatry fellowship. Dr. Hanson would also like to thank the psychology staff of the Maryland Reception Diagnostic and Classification Center for their help and friendship over the last twenty years. We've survived some amazing times. Dr. Daviss would also like to acknowledge Colleen Roach, R.N., Larry Linder, M.D., and Jim Walker, whose support at the Baltimore Washington Medical Center has been unparalleled; Barbara Fowler, Ph.D., who puts up with his bad jokes and puns on a daily basis; his parents and family; his sister, Cindy McKinney; his ex-wife, Donna Kane; his son, Nathan Daviss, for his awesome artistic contributions; friend and colleague, Kim Solberg, M.D; and David A. Lewis, M.D., who taught him so much about brain research and writing. He also wants particularly to recognize Paul Mc-Clelland, M.D., who has been a special friend and mentor to him for over twenty years.

This book came about because of dialogue on the *Shrink Rap* blog and the *My Three Shrinks* podcast. Those who contributed to these efforts stimulated our thoughts, forced us to question our beliefs, and inspired us to see that there is a need for a book that explains what psychiatrists do. As we've thought about the book, we've posted our ideas on the blog and let our blog readers shape them. When we went to create the suggested reading section, we shamelessly asked our readers to contribute by telling us what books had inspired or helped them personally.

We'd like to thank our blog and podcast guests: Chris Kraft, Ph.D., Mark Komrad, M.D., J. Raymond DePaulo, M.D., Patrick Barta, M.D., Gariane Gunter, M.D., Peter V. Rabins, M.D., Ronald Pies, M.D., Mitchell Newmark, M.D., Gerald Klee, M.D., Eric Kuhn, Peter Owens, Ph.D., "Dr. Dave" Van Nuys from *Shrink Rap Radio* (a separate endeavor), and those who've contributed under pseudonyms, including Retriever, DoctorAnonymous, and CoveringDoc.

We'd also like to thank our many readers and listeners who've engaged with us and helped with this process, including (please forgive the oversight if we've left you out): AA, ABF, AJ, Alison Cummins, Ally, Anastacia, Andrea, Ania (a psychiatrist who learned from veterans), April, Aqua, Ariel, Attachment Girl, Barb, Barbara K., Bardiac, Battle Weary, Bee, Bippidee, Blogbehave, Butterfly, Camel, Catherine, Cheryl Fuller, Ph.D., Child Psych, ChristinePAS, CoachKiki, Crystal, Daniel Carlat, M.D., David Pogue, Denni, DK, Donna Garfield, Drytears, DoctorAnonymous, Dr. Bob, Dr. John Crippen, Dr. Pink Freud, Dr. Psychobabble, Dr. Rob, Dr. Shock, Dr. Val, Dr. X, Dragonfly, drdymphna, Dreaming again, DrivingMissMolly, d'Zhouy, EastCoaster, ELN, Emy L.

Nosti, Esther, Fat Doctor, Foofoo5, Fordo, Foveva, Gerbil, HappyOrganist, Health Psych, healthskills, itsjustme, ItsTheWooo, Ivory, Janie, Jayme, jcat, Jen, Jenny, Jessa, Jesse, JJ, John, Jonathan Schnapp, jstrong, JW, Karen, Karla, Kathy, Katie, KBAB, KevinMD, Kim, Ladyk73, Lee, Lisa, Lockup Doc, Lola Snow, Lu, Maggie, Marcia, Marie, Matt, Meg, Merope3, Michele, Michelle, Michreneeg, Midwife with a Knife, Mike, Mindful, Mind Hacks, mini UK, Miss Mouse, Momma, Mother Jones RN, Movie-Doc, Mr Ian, Mrs Cake, Murky Thoughts, Musings of a Dinosaur, Mysadalterego, Nardilfan, NeoNurseChic, neurocritic, nonstandard mind, Notfluffy, Novalis, nutty, OmniBrain, one4theroad, onelongjourney, on the same page, Optic1, Paperdoll, Patient Anonymous, Paula, Pemdas, Perished Core, Pete, Phoebe, Pleochroia, Prynne, Psychiatry101, Purplesque, QoS, Rach, Randall Sexton, Retriever, Return of Saturn, rlbates, Roia, Romeo Vitelli, Ronald Pies, M.D., Roses, rosysunset, Russell, Ruth, S, Sandy Ph.D., Sara, Sarah, Sarebear, Sasha8988, savantdanish, Scream, Sherri, shiny happy person, shrinkrapradio, ShrinkWife, Shruti, Si, Sophizo, Spiritual Emergency, Spiritual Recovery, stevebMD, Still dreaming, Sue in N. Va, Sunny CA, Syna, T, talesofacrazypsychmajor, The Alienist, The Crazy Music Lady, The Girl, The Hyperlexian Aspie, the last psychiatrist, The Shrink, The Silent Voices in my Mind, theamazingworldofpsychiatry, themadandwild, therapydoc, TherapyPatient, Tigermom, Tracy, Trick Cycling for Beginners, Uma, Vicki, wetnurse, William, Woundedgenius, Yay, Zoe Brain, anonymous (all of them), and the dozens of podcast listeners who have taken the time to put reviews of *My Three Shrinks* up on iTunes or to write to us with questions.

All medical specialties involve consultation, and psychiatry is no exception. The following people have provided curbside consultation, intellectual stimulation and inspiration, friendship, and mentoring during this process: Sally Waddington, M.D., Jesse Hellman, M.D., Steven Crawford, M.D., Michael Richardson, M.D., Lisa Beasley, M.D., Roger Lewin, M.D., Jonas Rappeport, M.D., Robert Roca, M.D., Jerald Block, M.D., Nicholas P. Conti, LCSW-C, Michael Kaminsky, M.D., Barbara Wilkov, Roni Davidi, Kathleen Sweeney, Carol Silberstein, the staff of the Maryland Psychiatric Society (Kery Hummel, Heidi Bunes, and Meagan Floyd), and the members and leaders of the Maryland Psychiatric Society. Frank Mondimore, M.D., and Danny Carlat, M.D., provided guidance as psychiatrist-authors. Our copy editor, Melanie Mallon, was patient through countless four-way discussions on the proper use of italics, hyphens, and the past perfect tense.

To our colleagues at the Johns Hopkins Community Psychiatry Program, Health Care for the Homeless, the Pro Bono Counseling Project, Baltimore Washington Medical Center, Greater Baltimore Medical Center, the Maryland Psychiatric Research Center, the Western Psychiatric Institute and Clinic, URAC, CCHIT's Behavioral Health Work Group, the American Psychiatric Association, and the Clifton T. Perkins Hospital Center, we thank you for giving us a more complete view of psychiatry's possibilities and limitations.

Finally, we'd like to thank the folks at the Johns Hopkins University Press for taking on this somewhat-less-than-conventional endeavor, and especially our amazing editor and sometimes referee, Jacqueline Wehmueller, whose insight, patience, kindness, and friendship have approached heroic proportions.

The most important influences for all three of us, more than any of the above, have been our patients. They are our most savvy and insightful teachers and know more about their mental health and illness than we ever could. This book is dedicated to them.

—The Shrink Rappers

Sources and Suggested Reading

Some of the resources listed here are materials that we have found helpful in our work or that our patients have found useful. Some books were recommended by trusted colleagues. In addition, we asked the readers of our Shrink Rap blog to tell us what books they have found helpful, and we include many of their recommendations here.

Other resources listed here were sources for information included in this book. In a more scholarly book, these works would be cited in footnotes, but we have chosen to weave our recommended readings and our sources together in one place.

Note: For the longer web links (URLs), we include within brackets a shorter bit.ly version to make it easier to type the link into your browser. For example, the short link to our blog post about our readers' favorite mental health books is http:// bit.ly/99yzxy. An updated list of this section, with clickable links, can be found at http://bit.ly/shrinkyreading.

Coping with Adversity

Viktor E. Frankl, *Man's Search for Meaning* (Boston: Beacon Press, 1968).

Forensic Psychiatry

Advance Directives: www.nrc-pad.org/index.php
America's Law Enforcement and Mental Health Project (Public Law 106-515), 1999–2000, bill text at http://thomas.loc.gov/cgi-bin/query/z?c106:S.1865. ENR: [*http://bit.ly/adtQgh*]

Paul Appelbaum and Tom Gutheil, *Clinical Handbook of Psychiatry and the Law* (Philadelphia: Lippincott Williams and Wilkins, 2006).

Canterbury v. Spence, 464 F.2d 772 (D.C. Cir. 1972)

John S. Goldkamp and Cheryl Irons-Guynn, *Emerging Judicial Strategies for the Mentally Ill in the Criminal Caseload: Mental Health Courts in Fort Lauderdale, Seattle, San Bernardino, and Anchorage.* Bureau of Justice Assistance Monograph, April 2000, NCJ 182504.

Kansas v. Crane, 534 U.S. 407 (2002)

Kansas v. Hendricks, 521 U.S. 346 (1997)

The MacArthur Coercion Study, May 2004, www.macarthur.virginia.edu/coercion.html [*http://bit.ly/b1EnhD*]

Gary Melton, John Petrila, Norman Poythress, and Christopher Slobogin, *Psychological Evaluations for the Courts* (New York: Guilford Press, 2007).

Pearson v. Probate, 309 U.S. 270 (1940)

Richard Rosner, ed., *Principles and Practice of Forensic Psychiatry* (New York: Oxford University Press; A Hodder Arnold Publication, 2003).

Diane Schetky and Elissa Benedek, *Clinical Handbook of Child Psychiatry and the Law* (Philadelphia: Williams and Wilkins, 1992).

Essi Viding, R. James Blair, Terrie Moffitt, and Robert Plomin, "Evidence for Substantial Genetic Risk for Psychopathy in 7-Year-Olds." *Journal of Child Psychology and Psychiatry* 46 (2005): 592–97.

The Future of Psychiatry

Steven R. Daviss, "Six Future Trends in Psychiatry," Shrink Rap Blog, February 20, 2009, http://psychiatrist-blog.blogspot.com/2009/02/six-future-trends-in-psychiatry.html [*http://bit.ly/uKxCl*]

P. Fitzgerald, "Brain Stimulation Techniques for the Treatment of Depression and Other Psychiatric Disorders." *Australasian Psychiatry* 16 (2008): 183–90.

Charles F. Reynolds III, David A. Lewis, et al., "The Future of Psychiatry as Clinical Neuroscience." *Academic Medicine* 84 (2009): 446–50. [*http://bit.ly/dsKjL5*]

Hospital-based Psychiatry

CCHIT, or Certification Commission for Health Information Technology, http://cchit.org

EMTALA, or Emergency Medical Treatment and Labor Act, www.cms.gov/EMTALA

A Declaration of Health Data Rights, www.Healthdatarights.org

HIPAA, or Health Insurance Portability and Accountability Act, www.hhs.gov/ocr/privacy

HITshrink Blog, http://hitshrink.blogspot.com

Joint Commission National Quality Core Measures—Hospital-Based Inpatient Psychiatric Services (HBIPS) Core Measure Set, www.jointcommission.org/hospital-based_inpatient_psychiatric_services/ [*http://bit.ly/fTjWhe*]

ONCHIT, or Office of the National Coordinator for Health Information Technology, http://healthit.hhs.gov

Physician Order Entry Team, Computerized Physician Order Entry, Oregon Health Sciences University, www.cpoe.org

Steven S. Sharfstein, Faith B. Dickerson, and John M. Oldham, *Textbook of Hospital Psychiatry* (Washington, DC: American Psychiatric Publishing, 2009).

Speak Flower, Speakflower.org

Illness and Occupation

Jonathan R. T. Davidson, Kathryn M. Connor, and Marvin Swartz, "Mental Illness in U.S. Presidents between 1776 and 1974: A Review of Biographical Sources." *Journal of Nervous and Mental Disease* 194 (2006): 47–51.

Medicine in General

Jerome Groopman, *How Doctors Think* (New York: Houghton Mifflin, 2007).

Pharmaceutical Company Influence

American Medical Association, "Ethical Guidelines for Gifts to Physicians from Industry." Accessed at www.ama-assn.org/ama/pub/physician-resources/medical-ethics/about-ethics-group/ethics-resource-center/educational-resources/guidelines-gifts-physicians.shtml [*http://bit.ly/8Z6UkG*]

Daniel J. Carlat, *Unhinged: The Trouble with Psychiatry: A Doctor's Revelations about a Profession in Crisis* (New York: Simon and Schuster, 2010).

Gardiner Harris, "Crackdown on Doctors Who Take Kickbacks," *New York Times*, March 3, 2009.

Gardiner Harris, "Document Details Plan to Promote Costly Drug," *New York Times*, September 1, 2009.

Jeanne Steiner, Michael Norko, Susan Devine, et al., "Best Practices: Developing

Ethical Guidelines for Pharmaceutical Company Support in an Academic Mental Health Center." *Psychiatric Services* 54 (2003): 1079–89.

Psychiatry in General

Daniel J. Carlat, *The Psychiatric Interview: A Practical Guide,* 2nd ed. (Philadelphia: Lippincott Williams and Wilkins, 2004).

E. Torrey Fuller, K. Entsminger, J. Geller, J. Stanley, D. J. Jaffe, "The Shortage of Public Hospital Beds for Mentally Ill Persons, A Report of the Treatment Advocacy Center," accessed at www.treatmentadvocacycenter.org/storage/tac/documents/the_shortage_of_publichospital_beds.pdf [*http://bit.ly/aQKOyd*]

Robert Klitzman, *In a House of Dreams and Glass: Becoming a Psychiatrist* (New York: Simon and Schuster, 1995).

Paul R. McHugh and Philip R. Slavney, *The Perspectives of Psychiatry,* 2nd ed. (Baltimore: Johns Hopkins University Press, 1998).

My Three Shrinks Podcast, http://mythreeshrinks.com

Shrink Rap Blog, http://psychiatrist-blog.blogspot.com

Charles F. Zorumski and Eugene Rubin, *Demystifying Psychiatry: A Resource for Patients and Families* (New York: Oxford University Press, 2009).

Psychoanalysis

Patrick Casement, *Learning from the Patient* (New York: Guilford Press, 1991).

Fred M. Levin, *Psyche and Brain: the Biology of Talking Cures* (International Universities Press, 2004).

Janet Malcolm, *Psychoanalysis: The Impossible Profession* (New York: Knopf, 1981).

Irvin Yalom, *Lying on the Couch: A Novel* (New York: Basic Books, 1996).

Psychotherapy

Michael Franz Basch, *Understanding Psychotherapy: The Science behind the Art* (New York: Basic Books, 1988).

Judith S. Beck, *Cognitive Therapy: Basics and Beyond* (New York: Guilford Press, 1995).

Glen O. Gabbard, *Principles of Psychodynamic Psychotherapy* (Washington, DC: American Psychiatric Publishing, 2009).

Glen O. Gabbard, *Textbook of Psychotherapeutic Treatments* (Washington, DC: American Psychiatric Publishing, 2008).

T. Byram Karasu, *Wisdom in the Practice of Psychotherapy* (New York: Basic Books, 1992).

Peter D. Kramer, *Should You Leave?* (New York: Scribner, 1997).

Deborah A. Lott, *In Session: The Bond between Women and Their Therapists* (New York: W.H. Freeman, 1999).

Jan Scott, J. Mark G. Williams, and Aaron T. Beck, *Cognitive Therapy in Clinical Practice: An Illustrative Casebook* (New York: Routledge, 1989).

Susan C. Vaughan, *The Talking Cure: The Science behind Psychotherapy* (New York: Putnam, 1997).

Irvin D. Yalom, *Existential Psychotherapy* (New York: Basic Books, 1980).

Irvin D. Yalom, *The Gift of Therapy: An Open Letter to a New Generation of Therapists and Their Patients* (New York: HarperCollins, 2002).

Irvin D. Yalom, *Love's Executioner and Other Tales of Psychotherapy* (New York: Basic Books, 1989).

Irvin D. Yalom and Ginny Elkin, *Every Day Gets a Little Closer: A Twice-Told Therapy* (New York: Basic Books, 1974).

Psychotropic Medications

Peter D. Kramer, *Listening to Prozac* (New York: Viking, 1993).

Alan F. Schatzberg, Jonathan O. Cole, and Charles Debattista, *Manual of Clinical Psychopharmacology*, 7th ed. (Washington, DC: American Psychiatric Publishing, 2010).

Stephen M. Stahl, *Stahl's Essential Psychopharmacology*, 3rd ed. (New York: Cambridge University Press, 2008).

Relationships and Communication

John Gottman, *The Seven Principles for Making Marriage Work* (New York: Crown, 1999).

Gordon Livingston, *How to Love* (New York: De Capo, 2009).

Harriet Lerner, *The Dance of Anger: A Woman's Guide to Changing the Patterns of Intimate Relationships* (New York: HarperCollins, 1985).

Harriet Lerner, *The Dance of Intimacy* (New York: HarperCollins, 1989).

M. Scott Peck, *The Road Less Traveled: A New Psychology of Love, Traditional Values and Spiritual Growth*, 25th anniversary edition (New York: Touchstone, 2003).

Douglas Stone, Bruce Patton, Sheila Heen, and Roger Fisher, *Difficult Conversations: How to Discuss What Matters Most* (New York: Viking Adult, 1999).

Specific Disorders

Edmund J. Bourne, *The Anxiety and Phobia Workbook*, 4th ed. (Oakland, CA: New Harbinger, 2005).

David D. Burns, *Feeling Good: The New Mood Therapy*, Revised and Updated (New York: Avon, 1999).

Lana R. Castle, *Bipolar Disorder Demystified: Mastering the Tightrope of Manic Depression* (New York: Marlowe, 2003).

J. Raymond DePaulo and Leslie Alan Horvitz, *Understanding Depression: What We Know and What You Can Do About It* (New York: Wiley, 2002).

Jerome D. Frank and Julia B. Frank, *Persuasion and Healing: A Comparative Study of Psychotherapy*, 3rd ed. (Baltimore: Johns Hopkins University Press, 1991).

Dan Frosch, "States Differ on Marijuana for PTSD," *New York Times*, March 24, 2010.

Marc Galanter and Herbert D. Kleber, *Textbook of Substance Abuse Treatment*, 4th ed. (Washington, DC: American Psychiatric Publishing, 2008).

Frederick K. Goodwin and Kay Redfield Jamison, *Manic-Depressive Illness: Bipolar Disorders and Recurrent Depression*, 2nd ed. (New York: Oxford University Press, 2007).

Marya Hornbacher, *Wasted: A Memoir of Anorexia and Bulimia* (New York: HarperCollins Publishers, 1998).

Kay Redfield Jamison, *Night Falls Fast: Understanding Suicide* (New York: Knopf, 1999).

Kay Redfield Jamison, *An Unquiet Mind: A Memoir of Moods and Madness* (New York: Knopf, 1995).

Nancy I. Mace and Peter V. Rabins, *The 36 Hour Day: A Family Guide to Caring for Persons with Alzheimer's Disease, Related Dementing Illnesses, and Memory Loss in Later Life,* 4th ed. (Baltimore: Johns Hopkins University Press, 2006).

James F. Masterson, *The Search for the Real Self: Unmasking the Personality Disorders of Our Age* (New York: Free Press, 1988).

Francis Mark Mondimore, *Bipolar Disorder: A Guide for Patients and Families,* 2nd ed. (Baltimore: Johns Hopkins University Press, 2006).

Francis Mark Mondimore, *Depression: The Mood Disease*, 3rd ed. (Baltimore: Johns Hopkins University Press, 2006).

Jim Phelps, *Why Am I Still Depressed? Recognizing and Managing the Ups and Downs of Bipolar II and Soft Bipolar Disorder* (New York: McGraw-Hill, 2006).

D. Robinson, M. Woerner, J. Alvir, et al., "Predictors of Relapse Following Response from a First Episode of Schizophrenia or Schizoaffective Disorder." *Archives of General Psychiatry* 56 (1999): 241–47.

Jenni Schaefer and Thom Rutledge, *Life without ED: How One Woman Declared Independence From Her Eating Disorder and You Can Too* (New York: McGraw-Hill, 2004).

Susan Sheehan, *Is There No Place on Earth for Me?* (New York: Vintage, 1982).

Deborah Sichel and Jeanne W. Driscoll, *Women's Moods: What Every Woman Must Know about Hormones, the Brain, and Emotional Health* (New York: William Morrow, 1999).

Andrew Solomon, *The Noonday Demon: An Atlas of Depression* (New York: Scribner, 2001).

William Styron, *Darkness Visible: A Memoir of Madness* (New York: Random House, 1990).

M. Zanarini, L. Barison, F. Frankenburg, et al., "Family History Study of the Familial Coaggregation of Borderline Personality Disorder with Axis I and Nonborderline Dramatic Cluster Axis II Disorders." *Journal of Personality Disorders* 23 (2009): 357–69.

About the Authors

Starting with Dinah Miller:

In the fall of 2005, I spent two weeks in Louisiana working as a volunteer psychiatrist with the Katrina Assistance Project. I came back feeling edgy, fragile, and powerless, all too aware that the world can be changed in a day by forces beyond us. I did what I do when I get edgy: I wrote about my experience. I finished an article about the journey, and it was time to move on. Still, I stayed fragile for a while, and I'm not sure why. Perhaps I'm remembering it all wrong. After all, my own life was intact, and I'd always known that all it takes to transform that serenity is one small jilt of the earth, one burst blood vessel, one evil terrorist, one moment of hesitation when pushing for the brake pedal. Hurricane Katrina didn't douse my home or uproot my family, though after seeing it up close, it felt a little more personal than the rest of the world's tragedies, and somehow that's where this story starts in my mind.

It was a hard winter. Work felt hard. My psychiatric patients were struggling, and I, as their doctor, was distracted. At first I couldn't write, and then I couldn't stop writing. I resumed the novel I'd begun the summer before. By spring, I finished another novel and saved it on my hard drive. My good friend Anne Hanson told me that doctors see tragedies all the time and that the distress and distraction I felt needed more of an explanation. I know what I felt. I don't know why.

I decided I wanted a blog. I'd never read a blog, and I wasn't really sure what one was, but whatever it was, I wanted it. I knew it would be a place to post my writing on the Internet, and that sounded good. I looked at

Michelle Malkin's political blog. I still didn't know what a blog was, and I still wanted one.

I called Anne Hanson and Steve Daviss, the coauthors of this book, who are both computer savvy, which is a nice way of saying that these two wonderful people are geeks. They initially grumbled, but they agreed to "help" me, and we spent the better part of a weekend setting up *Shrink Rap*.

Shrink Rap seized me, and my two friends quickly became engrossed as enthusiastic co bloggers. They insisted, however, on remaining anonymous because it was the only way they could feel free to write about their work, and so "Roy" and "ClinkShrink" were born.

There was a time long before *Shrink Rap* when Steve asked if I wanted to join LinkedIn, an online networking site. "Why would I want to talk to people I don't know?" I had asked. Funny, but now I talk to people I don't know all the time on our blog. Readers comment on our posts, and we respond. They tell us about their lives, their experience as therapists, and more often, their experience as psychiatric patients. One lovely nurse in Philadelphia sends us e-mails with her piano music, and when she had a fender bender, she managed to get a photo of her car linked into the comment section of *Shrink Rap*. In case my real life, with all its family and professional demands, wasn't enough, I now have a virtual life, too.

Steve insisted we needed a podcast to go with *Shrink Rap*. I didn't know what a podcast was, and I didn't particularly want one, but Steve walked us through the production of many episodes of *My Three Shrinks*, and that's how I learned. We're proud to say that ours is one of the most popular psychiatry podcasts on the web, and we hope you'll visit iTunes or MyThreeShrinks.com to listen to us chat. We've had some terrific and prestigious guests join us, and now we have our own niche on the web.

I started *Shrink Rap* because I wanted a forum to express some of my thoughts about my experience of psychiatry. Some days things are pretty serious, and other days they are a bit more whimsical. My dog's picture has been posted; we've adopted the duck as our blog mascot; and Steve woke up in the middle of the night once and wrote about his dreams. Anne likes to talk about her adventures as a rock climber and nature and chocolate, when she's not talking about her work as a forensic psychiatrist in the correctional system.

Shrink Rap turned out to be more fun than I ever imagined it would be. My friendships with Anne and Steve—two delightful and brilliant people—have grown deeper, and our lives now frequently intertwine both on and off the Internet. I've enjoyed "meeting" the readers who engage us in both intellectual and entertaining conversations. The biggest surprise, however, has not been what we've learned from talking with other mental health professionals, but the insights we've gained from patients who share their inner worlds with us in a way that patients often hide from their real-life psychiatrists. In so many ways, this has been an educational process that can't be had in any other forum.

This book was conceived as a way to share the *Shrink Rap* and *My Three Shrinks* experience with a broader audience and to include those who might like a glimpse at how psychiatrists think without either stumbling upon us on the Internet or weaving through the thousands of pages of blog material and hours upon hours of podcasts that have now been produced. Certainly, we invite you to visit us in those forums, but this is an effort to present our expertise and professional dynamics in a more concise and organized way.

Just a quick word about who I am and what I do. I am a general adult outpatient psychiatrist. I have a private psychotherapy practice, and I prescribe medications when needed, which is often. I have also worked in three community mental health centers in the Baltimore area, and since 1998, I've worked at the Johns Hopkins Community Psychiatry Program. For many years, I was a consultant to the Johns Hopkins Sexual Behaviors Consultation Unit. In clinic settings, I work with chronically mentally ill and indigent patients who cannot access private care. I have worked in a number of administrative and supervisory capacities, and during the year we wrote this book, I was president of the Maryland Psychiatric Society. And in case I forgot to mention it, I love to write.

Next up is Steve Daviss:
That's pretty much the way I remember it, too. Dinah wanted a blog, and somehow it became my problem: "I don't know what one is or how to do it, but I want one." She wanted to write and have an immediate audience, even if it was just one person in Vanuatu.

I first met Dinah about thirteen years ago at a community mental health center, where I worked for a few hours a week, and she was the medical director. After we both left that clinic, we occasionally ran into each other. When her blogging inspiration hit, I agreed to write some blog posts on psychopharmacology, pharmacogenetics, and other psychiatric areas that I think about.

I have six or seven family members who have mental illness and grew up wondering how such a thing could happen. I initially went to medical school to learn more about the brain and body, because I wanted to go into research. After completing a schizophrenia research fellowship at the Maryland Psychiatric Research Center, where I did postmortem brain research, I realized how much I missed clinical care. I have since worked in community mental health clinics, private practice, nursing homes, addiction programs, hospitals, and emergency departments. I am a past president of the Maryland Psychiatric Society, a Distinguished Fellow of the American Psychiatric Association, and have volunteered for the insurance accrediting body URAC and for the Certification Commission for Health Information Technology (CCHIT), where I served as the co-chair of the Behavioral Health Work Group, and for the Maryland Health Care Commission's Health Information Exchange Policy Board.

I like to educate people, to explain things so that others understand how I came to the conclusion I did, and *Shrink Rap* quickly became a place to do this. Psychiatry is, unfortunately, a misunderstood field, particularly as it intersects the broader field of medicine. One goal of this book is to open a window into our collective brain so that you can see what goes into the decision-making process for a psychiatrist. At *Shrink Rap*, we've been able to demystify it while also meeting our own needs for a creative outlet. Some might simply say I have a pathological need to inflict my bad puns on others! Finally, I love hearing others' perspectives on issues that are important to me, especially folks from other countries, and *Shrink Rap* has a worldwide readership.

So, that's what I got out of *Shrink Rap*. But, I wanted something more, so I pushed for the podcast. Unlike Dinah, I knew what a podcast was, I knew we had to have one, and so *My Three Shrinks* was born on December 4, 2006. There was already a talk radio show and podcast called *Shrink Rap Radio*, so we came up with *My Three Shrinks*. I designed the logo after the three sets of animated feet from the 1960s TV sitcom *My Three Sons*. (Has anyone figured out whose feet are whose yet?)

We started out recording it with a Snowball USB mic from Blue for $99. It was acceptable, but I spoke louder than Dinah and Anne, so the sound quality varied. It also picked up a lot of background noise, like the bus down the street and the refrigerator in Dinah's kitchen. Around podcast #38 or so, we decided to get a better audio setup, so Dinah sprung for a soundboard and individual condenser microphones. That really made a big difference and provided a more professional polish. Yes, we do it for fun, and some of the creative part with this, for me, is the tech side, tweaking things here and there, adding new doodads and such. I am very much a numbers person, so I love to analyze numbers and patterns and find hidden relationships, which you will understand from my writing.

Dinah kept pushing us to do a book together, because numerous readers and listeners gave us ego-inflating compliments about how educational and entertaining we were. One iTunes reviewer wrote, "If you have any interest in the realm of psychiatry then you must listen to this podcast. Dinah, ClinkShrink and Roy do a wonderful job of presenting psychiatric issues in layman's terms that are both easy to understand and hilarious to listen to. . . . It's like going to med school, minus all the studying plus a whole lot cheaper."

I think it is the playful interaction among the three of us that provides our secret sauce. We've toned down some of our "witty banter" for our book but hope to help the reader see how psychiatrists think about different issues in mental health and how it is we agree and disagree, and to provide some insight into what psychiatry is all about. Or, at least, what it is about for these three docs.

You learned that Dinah is the outpatient psychiatrist with the psychotherapy practice. I am the consultation-liaison psychiatrist. What's that? A consultation-liaison (C-L) psychiatrist works in a general hospital setting, providing consultations to medical colleagues on their patients who are admitted to regular medical-surgical inpatient units. I see the people who hallucinate after surgery, or get manic on prednisone, or are depressed after a heart attack, or take an overdose of medications. My job is to figure out what is wrong and how to make things better. I sometimes see people in the Emergency Department for similar problems, too. I am currently the department chair for psychiatry at Baltimore Washington Medical Center. I like the more biological side of psychiatry, such as psychopharmacology, pharmacogenetics, and clinical informatics. In fact, I am now pursuing my second career in clinical informatics and hope to work as a chief medical information officer at a hospital or a tech company next.

And finally, Anne Hanson:
When Dinah asked me to help with her blog, my first thought was, "Oh dear. I'm going to get fired." You see, I work in a prison as a forensic psychiatrist, which means that I work with mentally ill people who are involved in the criminal justice system. Forensic psychiatrists also do court-ordered psychiatric evaluations, and they testify about civil issues like malpractice and child custody. I've done that in the past, but right now my forensic work is entirely in a correctional system. Correctional facilities are jails or prisons and are notoriously defensive and secretive systems, so I didn't think prison officials would look too kindly on my blogging about my work there.

I thought about this and weighed it against the fact that the general public may not be aware of the amount of health care that is provided to prisoners. They also may not know too much about what life inside a correctional facility is like, aside from what they've seen in television shows and in movies like *The Green Mile*. I wanted to educate people, and I wanted a chance to challenge and correct stereotypes and to explain in more detail what it is that I do. And so I began blogging.

I enjoy my time blogging with Dinah and Steve. They are both very articulate and smart people, and they're fun to argue with. Forensic psychiatrists like to debate about things, thus the attraction to legal issues. When I write I often focus on issues related to case law as well as health care costs and access to treatment. My work in prison has made me very aware of the distinctions between the haves and have-nots of society, and I tend to get on a soapbox about this. Fortunately, Dinah and Steve are patient with me.

When people read this book, my hope is that they will remember what I've written the next time they have to vote about providing money for correctional facilities, correctional health care, or the public mental health system. I hope they remember the hidden world that goes on every day behind bars and the people we have an obligation to care for there.

Besides working with prisoners, I am the director of the forensic psychiatry fellowship at the University of Maryland. I enjoy my role as educator, and I hope this book educates the public about psychiatrists and the patients for whom we provide care.

Dinah, Steve, and I hope you will enjoy reading this book as much as we enjoyed writing it. If you'd like to join our continuing conversation, please feel free to visit us online, at *Shrink Rap* and at *My Three Shrinks*.

Index

abnormal movements, in physical exam, 26

activation syndrome, 114

actus reus, 146

acuity level, in hospital inpatient unit, 161

ADA. *See* Americans with Disabilities Act

addiction, 53–56; and anxiety, 86, 215–16; to pornography, 52–54; and prescription medications, 214–17; red flags for, 216; reimbursement for treatment of, 206; and Xanax, 93–96

adjudicated delinquent, 130

adolescents. *See* children and adolescents

advance directives in psychiatry, 124

adverse effects. *See* side effects

age of consent, for treatment of minors, 127

alcoholism. *See* addiction

alprazolam. *See* Xanax

alternative medicine, 217–18

alters, in multiple personality disorder, 106

American Foundation for Suicide Prevention, 59

American Law Institute (ALI), test for insanity defense, 148

Americans with Disabilities Act (ADA), 210

Amplichip P450 (Roche), pharmaco-genetic test, 224–25

animals, for emotional support, 211

antianxiety medications, and addiction, 86, 214–17

antidepressants: dosing of, 90–91; effect on hippocampus, 224; suicidal thoughts caused by, 112–16

antipsychiatry movement, 219

antipsychotics: side effects of, 116; weight gain with, 111, 116

antisocial personality disorder (ASPD), 50–51; comorbidity in, 146; described in DSM, 144; genetic component in, 145. *See also* sociopaths

anxiety. *See* antianxiety medications

asthma, and mania, 25, 34

augmentation, of medications, 91

Ayurvedic medicine, 218

bed registry, central, 162

behavior: compulsive, 53–56; normal vs. pathological, 206–8

benefit-risk analysis. *See* risk-benefit analysis

benzodiazepines, 93–97, 214–17; withdrawal from, 94–95

biological factors, in psychiatric disorders, 30

bipolar disorder, 97; and borderline personality disorder, 206; diagnosis of, 208; and family history, 31; rapid-cycling type, 109; treatment by psychiatrist for, 14; types I and II, 109; Zoloft and, 33–34

black box warning, 112–15

borderline personality disorder, 49–50; and bipolar disorder, 206

boundaries: physician self-disclosure, 118; rules for maintaining, 118–19; treatment fees and, 119; violations of, 105, 118–21

brain: imaging: 165, 221–22; mapping, 222; maturation of frontal lobes and suicide risk, 115

Bush, George W., and NHIN, 175

Canterbury v. Spence, 88

carbamazepine, 111

Certification Commission for Health Information Technology (CCHIT), 177

certification criteria, for involuntary hospitalization, 164

chemical imbalance, explanation of, 29–31

children and adolescents: at-risk children, 126; emancipation of, 128; mandatory reporting laws for abuse of, 128; neglect, 126; remediation plans in, 126; suicidal thoughts with SSRI antidepressants in, 113–15

chlorazepate, 93

chlordiazepoxide, 93, 214

chronic pain: DBS treatment of, 223; rTMS treatment of, 222

Church of Scientology, 219

civil commitment, 36–39; hearings for, 37; *parens patriae*, 36; police powers in, 36; in sex offenders, 154–57

Civil Rights for Institutionalized Persons Act (CRIPA), 40

clinicaltrials.gov, 114

clozapine, 111, 225

cognitive-behavioral psychotherapy, 65

collateral history, 28–29

commitment laws: inpatient, 36–39; outpatient, 159

commitment standard, 37–38; *Lessard v. Schmidt*, 37

compelled treatment, 138

competency: in juveniles, 131; and medical decisions, 123, 126, 128; to stand trial, 142

complementary medicine, 89–90, 217–18

compulsive behaviors, 53–56

compulsory treatment. *See* compelled treatment

computerized axial tomography (CT) scan, 221

computerized patient record. *See* electronic health record

conditional release, 149

conduct disorder, leading to antisocial personality disorder, 145

confidentiality: and EHRs, 176–79; and psychotherapy, 63, 74–78

consent: informed, 87–89, 105; by minors, 128

consultation-liaison psychiatry, 180–82, 243–44

continued stay authorization, 171

controlled substances, 92–97

controversies, 201–20

core measures, in hospitals, 169, 173–74

couch, 9–10

counselors, 9

court: *parens patriae* power, 125; remediation plan, 126; specialty, 136. *See also* mental health courts

court, types of: drug, 136; juvenile, 125, 129–30; mental health, 136–38

court-ordered treatment, 12

CRIPA. *See* Civil Rights for Institutionalized Persons Act

crisis beds, 172

CT scan. *See* computerized axial tomography scan

custody evaluations, 132; "best interests of the child" standard, 133–34

Daviss, Steven Roy, and FDA Advisory Committee on Psychopharmacology, 113

day hospitals, 179–80

DBS. *See* deep brain stimulation

Declaration of Health Data Rights, 177

deep brain stimulation (DBS), 92, 223

defective delinquent statutes, 155

defense mechanisms, 108

de-institutionalization movement, 172

delinquency: definition of, 130; proceedings in juvenile court, 129

delusions, 13, 161

depression: diagnostic criteria for, 31–33; effect of, on hippocampus, 224; major, 28; in prisoners, 151–52; suicidal thoughts in, 112–16; treatment-resistant type, 91, 222–23; vs. grief, 45

diabetes, drug-induced, 115–16

diagnosis: criteria for, in major depression, 32–33; and DSM, 204–6; impression, in psychiatric evaluation, 27; as label, 208; for research purposes, 205

diagnostic-related group (DRG), 182

Diagnostic and Statistical Manual of Mental Disorders (DSM), 31–33; antisocial personality disorder, 144; controversy over fifth edition, 204–8; DSM-II, 205; DSM-IV-TR, 31–33, 42; DSM-V, 31, 204; "psychopath" in, 144

diazepam, 93, 214

direct-to-consumer (DTC) marketing, 197

disability: and ADA, 210; benefits, 208–10

discharge planning, 172–74

disclosure. *See* self-disclosure

discrimination, in insurance, 189

disposition hearing, in juvenile court, 130

Dissociation (journal), 106

dissociative identity disorder (DID), 104, 106; diagnosis of, 208

Dix, Dorothea, 36, 127

DNA, in psychiatry, 224

doctor, defined, 8

dopamine receptor, 225

DRG. *See* diagnostic-related group

drug abuse. *See* addiction

drug companies. *See* pharmaceutical companies

drug interaction alerts, and EHR, 176

DSM. See *Diagnostic and Statistical Manual of Mental Disorders*

DTC marketing. *See* direct-to-consumer (DTC) marketing

ducks: as support animals, 211; in *Shrink Rap*, 240

Durham rule for insanity test, 148

Eagleton, Thomas, and stigma, 212

ECT. *See* electroconvulsive therapy

education, as part of treatment plan, 166

EHR. *See* electronic health record

electroconvulsive therapy (ECT), 91–92, 170

electromagnetic treatments. *See* treatments, electromagnetic

electronic health record (EHR), 174–79

emancipation of minors, 128

Emergency Department (ED), 6, 10–11, 35–36; decision to admit, 160; psychiatric evaluation in, 22, 159–64

Emergency Medical Treatment and Labor Act (EMTALA), 161–62

emergency petition, 36–37, 159

emergency room. *See* Emergency Department

emotional support animals, 211

e-patients, 177

expert witness, 12

FAA. *See* Federal Aviation Administration

family involvement, during hospitalization, 167

FDA. *See* Food and Drug Administration

Federal Aviation Administration (FAA), and pilots taking medications, 212

fees: for missed appointments, 190; for treatment, 185; waiving, 119, 195–96

fitness for duty, 212–13

fluoxetine, 30, 110; and suicidal thoughts, 112

fMRI. *See* functional MRI

follow-up care, in depression, 115

Food and Drug Administration (FDA), 112–16; Advisory Committee on Psychopharmacology, 113–15; black box warning, 112–15; labeling, 114; and pharmaceutical advertising, 197; and supplements, 90

forensic hospitals, 148, 172

forensic psychiatry, 12, 244; brain scans and, 222

functional MRI (fMRI), 221–22

GABA, 94

general hospital psychiatric units, 173

genetics, 30, 111, 224–25

genomic medicine, 224–25

genotype, 224

gifts, from patients, 198–99

Glenmullen, Joe *(Prozac Backlash),* 114

GNB3 gene, 111

Google Health, 176

grief, 45

group therapy, on hospital inpatient unit, 167

guardianship, and child welfare, 128. *See also* legal guardian

hallucinations, 13; brain mapping and, 222; and depression, 45

Hare Psychopathy Check List–Revised (PCL-R), 145

health care: proxy, 123; rationing, 202–3; reform, 202–4

healthdatarights.org, 177

Health Information Technology Policy Committee, 177

Health Insurance Portability and Accountability Act (HIPAA), 75, 176

herbal supplements, 89–90

hippocampus, 224

HITECH Act, 177

homosexuality, and DSM, 205–6

hospitals, 158–82; admission from ED, 160–61; day, 179–80; EMTALA, 161–62; forensic, 148; inpatient, 164–75, 203; long-term, 172–73; and managed care, 203; outpatient clinics, 180; psychiatric evaluation in,

22, 180–81; state psychiatric, 127; teaching, 22, 180; transfers between, 160, 163

impulsiveness, decreasing with age, 115
incompetency. *See* competency
informed consent, 87–89, 105; for medications, 192
inpatient. *See* hospitals, inpatient
insanity defense, 143, 147–49
insurance: accepting assignment, 187; commissioner, 163; companies, 162–63, 165; malpractice, 191–93; and Mental Health Parity Act, 189; participation in, 184–85; preauthorization process, 187; and review process, 171; and split therapy, 186; usual and customary rate, 187
interrogation techniques, 140–41
involuntary commitment, 36–39, 159, 164
involuntary medication, 39
irresistible impulse test for insanity defense, 148

jail, 11–12; vs. prison, 149. *See also* prison
Joint Commission, 169, 173–74
juvenile justice system: delinquency proceedings in, 129; disposition hearings in, 130; juvenile courts, creation of, 125; rehabilitation facilities in, 130; status conferences in, 137; transfer of jurisdiction to/from, 130; waiver from, 130

Kansas v. Crane, 156
Kansas v. Hendricks, 155
Koch, J. L., coining of term "psychopath," 144

lab tests, 15, 27; 192; in hospital inpatient unit, 165; with lithium, 116
Lamictal (lamotrigine), 111
learning disabilities, 211
least restrictive environment, 172
legal, guardian, 123. *See also* forensic psychiatry
Librium, 93, 214
licensing boards, 109
lithium, 110, 116

MacArthur Foundation, landmark study on coerced treatment, 138
Magna Carta, role in changing interrogation techniques, 140
magnetic resonance imaging (MRI), 221
major depression, 28. *See also* depression
malpractice insurance, 191–93
managed care: and authorizations for treatment, 171, 187; and inpatient hospitalization, 203; intrusion into treatment process, 188
mandatory reporting laws for child abuse, 128
mania, 33–35; induction by antidepressants, 115
marijuana: abuse of, 28; medical use of, 216–17
material risk standard, for informed consent, 88
McNaughten test for insanity defense, 147–48
"meaningful use," 177
medical records: electronic, 174–79; and HIPAA, 176; right to review, 40
medical school, 8
medication management, 15, 63; reimbursement for, 185

medications: augmentation of, 91; classification of, 83; costs, 203; dosing of, 90–91; in emergencies, 168; informed consent for, 192; metabolism of, 96–97; off-label use of, 83; prescribing, 15, 84; prescribing in prisons, 152; and treatment planning, 166. *See also* antidepressants; antipsychotics; benzodiazepines; mood stabilizers; stimulants
memory loss, with ECT, 170
mens rea, 147
Mental Health America, 169
Mental Health Bell, 169
mental health courts: constitutionality of, 138; effectiveness of, 138; eligibility criteria for, 137; history of, 136–38
Mental Health Parity and Addiction Equity Act of 2008 (MHPAEA), 189
mental health professionals, 7–10. *See also* psychiatrists; psychoanalysts; psychologists; social workers; therapists
mental illness: definition of, 204–5; in presidents of the United States, 212, 213–14
methylphenidate, 214
Microsoft HealthVault, 176
milieu therapy, 167
Mini-Mental Status Exam (MMSE), 26–27
mirtazapine, 110
missed appointments, 190–91
Model Penal Code test for insanity defense, 148
mood stabilizers, 33–34
moral insanity, 144
MRI. *See* magnetic resonance imaging
multiple personality disorder, 104, 106; diagnosis of, 208
My Three Shrinks podcast, 242–43

Narcotics Anonymous, 54
National Association of State Mental Health Program Directors (NASMHPD), 156
National Center for Complementary and Alternative Medicine (NCCAM), 90, 218
National Health Information Network (NHIN), 175
National Resource Center on Psychiatric Advance Directives, 124
neurons, 223
neuroplasticity, 223–24
neurotransmitters, 30–31, 94
no-shows. *See* missed appointments
nursing assessment, in hospital inpatient unit, 165
nutritional supplements, 89–90

obesity, 111
obsessive-compulsive disorder (OCD), 54; treatment using DBS, 223
occupational therapists, 165
Office of the National Coordinator for Health Information Technology (ONCHIT or ONC), 177
off-label use of medications, 83
olanzapine. *See* Zyprexa
One Flew Over the Cuckoo's Nest, 170
Osheroff v. Chestnut Lodge, 108
out-of-network (insurance), 184–85, 188
outpatient treatment: clinics, 180; commitment, 38; psychiatric evaluation in, 21–22
overhead expenses, in private practice, 187

panic attacks, 68, 80–81
paraphilias: and DSM-V, 207; rejection of diagnosis, 156
parens patriae powers, 125
parental rights, 126, 128

parity, 189
Parkinson's disease, treatment using
DBS, 223
partial hospitalization program
(PHP), 179–80
past life regression, 107
patients: gift-giving, 118; phone calls,
101–2; setting limits, 101–3
Patriot Act, and confidentiality, 76–77
PCL-R. *See* Hare Psychopathy Check
List–Revised
PCP. *See* primary care physician
Pearson v. Probate, 155
personal health information (PHI),
and HIPAA, 176
personal health record (PHR), 176–77
personality disorders, 48–52
personalized medicine, 224–25
PET scan. *See* positron emission
tomography scan
P450 liver enzymes, 224–25
pharmaceutical companies, 114, 196–98
pharmacogenetics, 96–97; and risk of
side effects, 114
PHI. *See* personal health information
PHP. *See* partial hospitalization
program
PHR. *See* personal health record
physician-assisted suicide, 58
pilots, and medications, 212
political repression, and psychiatric
diagnosis, 207
pornography, addiction to, 52–54
positron emission tomography (PET)
scan, 221
preauthorizations, for insurance, 187, 203
prednisone, inducing mania, 34
prescribing, 15; in prison, 152
pretrial detainees, 149, 172
primary care physician (PCP), 13
prison, 12; creation of therapeutic,
154; difference between jail and,

149; prescribing medications in,
152; reception center, 149–50
prisoners: classification of, 153; and
intake procedures, 151; and medication choice, 152–53
Pritchard, James: and "moral insanity," 144; *Treatise on Insanity*, 143
privacy: and EHRs, 176–79; in psychotherapy, 74–78
private practice, 183–200; psychiatric
evaluation in, 22
product test for insanity defense, 148
professional degrees, 8–9; certification, 9; forensic, 12; licensure, 9
prospective review process, 171
Prozac, 30, 110; and suicidal thoughts,
112
Prozac Backlash (Glenmullen), 114
psychiatric evaluation, 21–29; chief
complaint, 23; collateral history,
28–29; in custody evaluations, 132;
family history, 24; forensic, 132;
history of present illness, 23; interview styles, 23–24; lab tests, 27, 30;
medical history, 25; mental status
exam, 26–27; past history, 25; social
history, 24; in various settings, 21–22
psychiatric units. *See* hospitals,
inpatient
psychiatrists: changing, 108–9; compared to PCPs, 13–14; consultation-
liaison (C-L), 123, 180–82, 243–44;
defined, 7–8; forensic, 12, 131, 150–51,
244; interview styles, 23–24; vs.
nonphysician therapists, 16–17;
prison work environment, 150;
psychotherapy, 16–18; theoretical
orientation, 23; training, 8
psychiatry: consultation-liaison (C-L),
180–82, 243–44; financial issues in
practicing, 184; future of, 221–26. *See
also* forensic psychiatry

psychoanalysis, 9–10, 64–65
psychoanalysts, 59; training, 10
"psychological parent," 133
psychological testing: in custody eval-
    uations, 133; in hospital inpatient
    unit, 165
psychologists, 8; on inpatient units,
    165; and prescribing, 15
psychopath, in DSM, 144. *See also*
    sociopaths
psychopathic personality statute, 155
psychopathy, 142–45
psychopharmacogenetics, 96–97
psychosomatic specialty. *See* psychia-
    try, consultation-liaison
psychotherapy, 59–60, 62–73; dura-
    tion of, 81; future of, 225–26; and
    gifts, 118; during inpatient hospital-
    ization, 167; self-disclosure, 118;
    split treatment, 15–18; supervision,
    60, 67; theory, rigid adherence to,
    107; training, 8; types, 64
psychotic disorder, 13

quiet room, 168–69

reasonable physician standard, for
    informed consent, 87
recovered memories, 104–5
recovery model, 219
reimbursement, 185–87
remediation plans, 126
Remeron, 110
repetitive transcranial magnetic stim-
    ulation (rTMS), 92, 222–23
repressed memories, 104–5
research, 69–70; and diagnosis, 205
restraints, physical, 41, 168–69
retrospective review process, 171
rights: in civil commitment, 37;
    CRIPA, 40; emancipation, 128;
    parental, 126, 128; patient, 40–41;

to personal health data, 176–77;
    privacy of minors, 128
risk-benefit analysis, 111; in black box
    warnings, 114; of antidepressants vs.
    suicide, 114; and prescribing addic-
    tive medications, 214–17; of using
    EHRs, 175–79
Ritalin, 214
Roche, 224
role induction, 71
rTMS. *See* repetitive transcranial
    magnetic stimulation

schizoid personality disorder, 49
schizophrenia, 225; risk of developing,
    206
seclusion, 168–69
security, and EHRs, 178
selective serotonin reuptake inhibitor
    (SSRI), 110; suicidal thoughts and,
    112–16
self-disclosure, in psychotherapy,
    77–80, 118
serotonin, 30–31; transporter, 225
sertraline: causing mania, 33–34; and
    suicidal thoughts, 112
sex offenders, 154–57; and commitment
    law, 157; cost of treatment, 156–57
sexual abuse, in childhood, 104–6
shock treatments, 170
Shrink Rap blog, 240–43
side effects of treatment, 99–121;
    agranulocytosis, 111; appetite
    increase, 110; DBS, 223; diabetes,
    109; kidney, 116; with lithium, 116;
    liver, 111, 116; with medications, 85,
    110–17; predicting, 225; prednisone,
    34; psychotherapy, 99; rare, 111–12;
    recovered memories, 105–6; rTMS,
    223; sedation, 110; sexual, 110; with
    steroids, 34; Stevens-Johnson syn-
    drome, 111; tardive dyskinesia, 111–12;

tremor, 110; VNS, 223; weight gain, 109–11; Zoloft, 33–34
social anxiety disorder, vs. shyness, 206
social reform movement, 127
Social Security benefits, 208–10
social workers, 8–9; in the ED, 160; in the inpatient unit, 165
sociopaths, 143–46; comorbidity in, 146; genetic component in, 145; history of, 143–44; neuroimaging studies in, 145; physiology of, 145; in prison, 194; treatment of, 145–46
SpeakFlower.org, 176
specialty courts. See courts, specialty; mental health courts
splitting, 50
split treatment: benefits of, 17–18; insurance reimbursement for, 186; risks of, 15–17
SSRI. See selective serotonin reuptake inhibitor
"stability," 14
standard of care, 108; FDA dictating, 115
state licensing boards, 109
state psychiatric hospitals: and forensic patients, 172–73; history of, 127; transfer to, 160–61
stem cells, 224
steroids, inducing mania, 34
Stevens-Johnson syndrome, 111
stigma, 60, 173, 178; disabilities and, 210–2; and DTC marketing, 197
stimulants, 214
"stress," as cause of symptoms, 44–48
suicidal ideation. See suicide, thoughts
suicide, 56–59; attempts, 14; risk assessment for, 193–94; risk factors, 58; risk in untreated depression, 114; thoughts, 102–3, 112–16; thoughts vs. behaviors, 114
suicidologists, 58

supervision, in psychotherapy, 60, 67
supportive psychotherapy, 65
symptoms: induced, 105; medications for, 110; normal vs. abnormal, 206–8; and stress, 44–48

tardive dyskinesia, 111–12
teenagers. See children and adolescents
Tegretol, 111
testimonial privilege, 75
therapists, 9; on hospital inpatient unit, 165
transcranial magnetic stimulation (TMS), 92, 222–23
transference, 9, 72–73
Tranxene, 93
trauma, 51–52
Treatise on Insanity (Pritchard), 143
treatment plan, 165–66
treatment-resistant depression. See depression, treatment-resistant type
treatments, electromagnetic, 222–23

usual and customary rate (UCR), 187

vagal nerve stimulation (VNS), 92, 223
Valium, 93, 214
violence, 194–95
VNS. See vagal nerve stimulation
vocational rehabilitation, 210–11

Wellstone-Domenici Act. See Mental Health Parity and Addiction Equity Act of 2008
withdrawal, from Xanax, 94–95

Xanax, 93–97, 214

Zoloft: causing mania, 33–34; suicidal thoughts and, 112
Zyprexa, and diabetes, 115